NATURAL RECIPES FOR

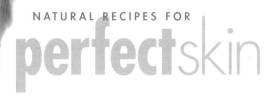

perfect skin

cosmetic masks
and lotions
that are good
enough to eat

Pierre Jean Cousin

D0543681

Quadrille

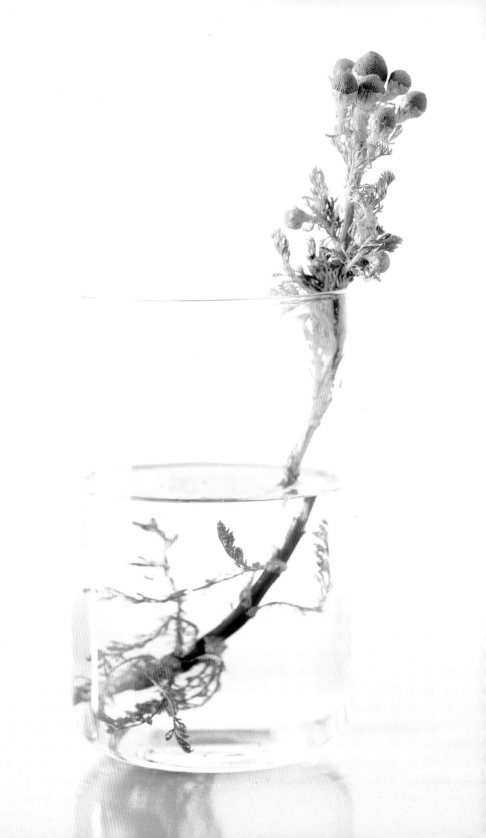

contents

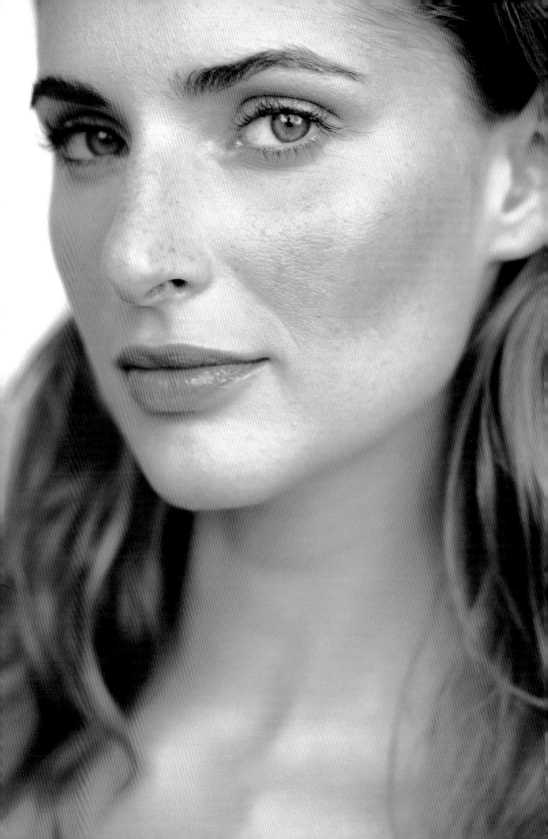

caring for your skin

Look at the skin on any part of your body under a microscope, and it will appear essentially the same. In spite of significant variations due to their particular function, the three layers of epidermis, dermis and hypodermis will always be visible.

The outer layer, or epidermis, is designed mainly to protect the active layer beneath and to regulate water evaporation. Composed of relatively hardwearing cells, it is subject to constant renewal as the dead, outermost cells are shed and replaced by new ones. It contains no blood vessels or nerve endings.

The layer beneath, the dermis, is the most hardworking and consequently responsible for most of the ageing process in skin. Its multiple functions of sensation, thermo-regulation, secretion and circulation require a complex structure made up of collagen, elastin, nerve endings, the upper parts of the sebaceous and sweat glands, and small blood vessels (or capillaries). Protein-based collagen fibres team up with elastin to create the elasticity in skin. The greatest concentrations of sebaceous glands occur in the scalp and around the forehead, mouth and nose, and their main function is to produce sebum, a lubricant indispensable for healthy skin and hair. Sweat glands eliminate toxins as well as regulate water levels in the body.

Below the dermis is the hypodermis, a layer of connective fatty tissues with a high water content. This contains the lower parts of the sebaceous and sweat glands, plus the hair follicles.

AGEING AND THE SKIN

Because we use the skin of the face to monitor changes in temperature and atmospheric conditions, and also, with facial muscle, as an important means of expression and communication, facial skin is naturally thinner and more sensitive than that on most other parts of our bodies. It is, therefore, on the face that the first signs of ageing in the skin appear. Yet the natural processes of deterioration caused by the passing years are at first invisible. By the time we reach adulthood the life-span of our skin cells has shortened dramatically: the average life of a skin cell in childhood is 100 days; for an adult it is about 50 days.

Aged 20–25 The earliest visible sign of ageing is likely to be the appearance of wrinkles. There are two kinds of wrinkles and they signal different stages in the process. The timing of their appearance is primarily determined by the genetic code, but it is accelerated by, in order of importance, sunlight, smoking, pollution and external factors such as wind, dryness, rapid changes of temperature or humidity, and dietary imbalance. Small, fine, mostly horizontal wrinkles appear first, initially as faint, occasional lines between the eyebrows and at the outer corners of the eyes. These are wrinkles of expression, and they are accentuated by laughing. Light freckles, if present, indicate over-exposure to the sun; they increase in number during the summer.

Between 25 and 35 More horizontal superficial lines of expression become visible now on the forehead and possibly around the mouth. The first lowering wrinkles may also appear – faint vertical lines between the outer edges of the nostrils and the corners of the mouth. These are the result of changes taking place in the hypodermis as gravity causes the fatty cells to migrate downwards. There is also a slight softening of the skin of the neck now, as it begins to lose some of its tone. Small, irregular, brown patches may appear as the skin pigments react to sudden over-exposure to sunlight.

By 40 Very gradually the wrinkles of expression and lowering are deepening and becoming permanent. Lack of skin tone in the neck increases, creating 'necklaces' of criss-crossing horizontal lines. The hypodermis of the neck has fewer of the fat cells and sebaceous glands necessary to keep the skin hydrated, and so, without adequate moisture, it is particularly vulnerable to the effects of ageing.

Between 45 and 55 By forty-five, the facial contours have begun to change as the bones thin and the skin loses some of its elasticity due to the disappearance of elastin in the dermis. In many cases the collagen is still intact, but the skin has already become softer and drier. The ability of the skin to retain water is greatly diminished – by up to one third if you compare the skin of a child with that of a mature adult. After the age of forty-five, the rate of ageing increases. The epidermis becomes thinner and, as the elastin continues to disappear, the collagen structure is disrupted, causing the dermo–epidermis junction to flatten. This is often vastly accelerated by lifestyle, in particular by smoking and prolonged exposure to sun. Changes in the hypodermis also speed up as the distribution of fatty tissues and fluid becomes more uneven and the effects of gravity increase the lowering process.

Between 55 and 65 A significant lowering of fatty tissues toward the chin and the lower jaw may change the shape of the face. Skin texture thickens on the face and neck. The disruption of collagen continues and the cells responsible for the restoration of elastin in the dermis disappear altogether.

After 65 As structural changes occur in the skin, its functions are also altered. The healing process takes longer, bruising becomes more frequent, waste products are eliminated more slowly, sensitivity is reduced and blood circulation is less efficient. In time, in consequence, the skin becomes more sensitive to infections and, finally, the production of vitamin D as well as the protection against the sun are impaired.

Ageing may be a genetically determined and essentially irreversible process, and it can be accelerated by chronic illnesses such as diabetes and atheroschlerosis, but it is important to eliminate any aggravating factors as far as possible to maintain and preserve the integrity of the three layers of the skin, both structurally and functionally.

Stress, pollution and changes in hormonal balance can all contribute to the premature ageing of the skin, but recent research shows that regular smokers invariably age far more quickly than non-smokers do. It is in the dermis that the damage is done. The elastin and collagen deteriorate faster, and vital supplies of oxygen and nutrients are reduced as nicotine contracts the capillaries to create grey, lifeless skin. Today, however, the skin's greatest enemy of all is the sun.

SUN AND THE SKIN

The most important external factor in the ageing of the skin is overexposure to the harmful rays of the sun. Some exposure to sunlight is beneficial – it stimulates the production of vitamin D, a substance essential for the formation and maintenance of healthy bones – but regular, prolonged sunbathing and exposure to ultraviolet rays is terribly destructive. And the dangers have increased considerably in recent years due to the destruction of the ozone layer.

There are two types of ultraviolet rays. UVB short-wave rays burn the two outer layers of the skin. Only 10 per cent of UVB rays reach the dermis, but they act upon the collagen–elastin association, causing its rapid and premature dissociation and significant loss of elasticity. Strongest at low latitudes and high altitudes, UVA long-wave rays are known to penetrate more deeply into the skin, contributing even more to the processes of wrinkling and loss of elasticity that result in ageing. Although UVB rays are thought to be responsible for sunburn and most skin cancers – more than 90 per cent of US skin cancers are attributed to UVB exposure – it is possible that UVA rays play some part in the causes of skin cancer.

Almost all sunscreens protect against UVB rays, but nothing is available to screen out all UVA rays. Even sunscreens offering a high sun protection factor (SPF) – a standard designed to measure a sunscreen's ability to protect the skin and prevent sunburn – leave your skin vulnerable to damage from UVA rays. Some researchers estimate that sunscreens advertising UVA protection are actually offering only SPF 3 or 4 protection against UVA rays; the higher stated SPF figure relates only to protection against UVB rays.

CHOOSING A SUNSCREEN

Of course, people burn at different rates, even within the same skin type, so you must decide if you are more or less sensitive to sun exposure and take appropriate measures. The advice is now widely available. Wear clothing that covers the body and shades the face. Apply an appropriate sunscreen to all exposed areas of the body, reapplying every two hours, even on cloudy days, and after swimming or perspiring. Minimise sun exposure between 10.00am and 3.00pm. Avoid unnecessary exposure to radiation through sun lamps or tanning parlours.

The table on the following page indicates the guidelines for minimum protection for all types of skin.

hair colour	skin colour	risk of freckles	risk of sunburn	tan type	recommended protection
white	albino	o	•••••	none; red sunburn with pain, swelling and peeling	sunblock
red	white	•••••	••••	as above	sunblock
fair	fair	••••	•••	very light after minor pink or red burns	sunblock
fair	fair	•••	••	light	SPF20–25
light brown	slightly dark	o	••	dark	SPF20–25
mid brown	slightly dark	o	•	dark	SPF15
dark brown	dark	o	o	very dark	SPF10
black	black	o	o	black	none

••••• = maximum risk   o = minimum risk   SPF30 = sunblock or absolute protection

Sunscreens with higher protection are helpful for those who want to reduce the risks still further, especially if they live or holiday at high altitudes, work outdoors, holiday at sea resorts, or perspire heavily. On holiday, for example, all fair-skinned people are recommended to use sunblock; people with slighter darker skin should use a sunblock or SPF30 for the first few days, followed by SPF25; dark-skinned people should use SPF20 with SPF25 on the shoulders and face.

To be on the safe side, always reduce by half the stated protection on any product. In reality a cream labelled Factor 10, for example, may for certain types of skin and in particular external conditions (such as wind, dilution of cream by salt water or heavy perspiration) offer only Factor 5 protection. Be aware also that SPF standards in the US are lower than those used in Europe, and that a tan is little protection from skin damage – it is reckoned to be equal to an SPF of 2.

SKIN TYPES

The first step in any personal natural skin-care programme is to establish which skin type you are. There are five basic groups, and a simple tissue test (see page 12) will establish to which you belong. It is worth doing this test even if you are confident of the result. Health, time, environment, even season, can cause temporary or permanent changes in skin condition. In fact, I recommend repeating the test every six months.

Normal skin Firm, supple, warm to the touch, neither dry nor greasy; without spots or blemishes. A pale normal skin will be pinkish. Normal skin is neither too acid nor too alkaline, with an average, neutral pH of 6.5.

Dry skin Dry (of course) and often slightly hot; prone to powdery scaling, superficial wrinkles and a dull appearance. This more acid type is sensitive to cold and wind, becoming irritated and inflamed, to central heating and to air conditioning. Moisturising is extremely important.

Oily skin Shiny and difficult to keep clean due to excess sebum (see page 6); frequent spots and inflamed areas, prone to acne and dermatitis. Sun, alcohol, poor diet, stress and cold damp winters aggravate the effects, but sebum inhibits water loss so this alkaline type can age slowly.

Combination skin Dry with shiny, oily areas on the forehead, sides of the nose, around the mouth and chin. Some areas need deep moisturising while others need astringent, drying applications.

Ageing skin Tending towards dryness, hot to touch and lacking tone or flexibility – a pinch will indicate how quickly it recovers; sometimes blemished, damaged or flushed with erythema (a hereditary redness due to the dilation of capillaries in the dermis). Ageing skin needs constant attention with toner, hydrating lotions and nourishing masks.

Two other skin types will be mentioned frequently: sensitive and damaged skin. 'Sensitive skin' is used to describe any skin type which responds especially quickly and adversely to sudden changes of temperature or humidity and bruises very easily; it is also allergic to many cosmetic products. A nightmare of a skin, it demands constant attention. 'Damaged skin' usually describes a localised area whose texture and/or appearance has changed due to a condition such as acne or eczema. Whether dry, oily or combination skin, damaged skin will exhibit some inflammation, scaling, thickening or scarring; special care is needed for these areas (see page 120).

THE TISSUE TEST

You need a completely clean face for this so remove any traces of makeup, and give your face a final clean, using warm water and cotton-wool balls. Gently towel dry and wait for about 30 minutes before covering your face with one ply (or layer) of a family-size paper tissue. Press lightly all over your face and leave for about 1 minute. Then remove the paper carefully and examine it near a window or a light.

Normal skin Faint oily traces on most of the paper.

Dry skin No oily traces: skin often becomes dry as it ages.

Oily skin Obvious oily stains over most of the paper.

Combination skin Oily patches at the sides of the nose and around the mouth and forehead.

BASIC SKIN CARE

The three important aspects of skin maintenance are well known and it is never too early to begin. Indeed, teenagers need to pay particular attention to their skin. A mild condition – a few spots, a small rash or eczema – can, if neglected, become severe, leading to scarring.

Cleansing Good cleansing removes the impurities, bacteria and dead cells that accumulate on the surface of the epidermis as well as any residue from makeup, while leaving as much of the lubricating natural oil (or sebum) as possible. A cleanser should therefore be gentle and natural. Unless your face is covered with mechanic's grease, there's no benefit in scrubbing with soap and water: harsh soaps and rubbing only strip the skin of vital oils and nutrients. A lotion is usually enough for daily cleansing. Once in a while, or on a more regular basis for those with oily skin, a clay, fruit or oat-based cleansing mask or some steaming should be used for a much deeper cleansing action.

Nourishing Dry and ageing skin in particular need additional oily substances, as well as minerals and small amounts of essential vitamins, to help maintain and regenerate normal vitality.

Toning Again, toning is particularly important in maintaining the elasticity of dry and ageing skin. However, it is vital to hydrate at the same time in order to maintain a normal level of fluid in the skin. It is for this reason that the natural toning recipes in this book combine astringents (to close the pores and reduce water loss) and moistening agents.

Some conventional skin-care programmes may present those three vital steps in a different order: cleanse, tone and then nourish. Natural-care programmes are based on the belief that it makes sense to close the pores after you feed the skin. So, for anyone who needs to nourish, remember the best routine: it's cleanse, nourish and then tone.

STARTING THE NATURAL SKIN-CARE PROGRAMME

Any of the recipes given in this book will fulfil at least one of these three tasks. Most of them offer a combination of beneficial actions. Once you have determined your skin type, you are ready to explore the recipe chapters. The summary at the foot of each recipe indicates the principle effects and appropriate skin types at a glance. Basic techniques are explained in more detail in the next chapter, including a section on massage and the application of essential oils (see pages 20–47), and there are other recipes to try there too. The book ends with a section devoted to common skin conditions, and here again there are programmes and additional recipes.

All the recipes are easy to prepare, but to make the most of them they must be applied regularly in a coherent skin-care programme. The following pages set out programmes for the basic skin types and for those with sensitive skin. Once you have established a workable routine, experiment by introducing other appropriate recipes and treatments – one at a time. You'll soon find out what works for you.

normal skin

teens

Use a gentle cleanser, such as a chamomile infusion (see page 30), daily. A cleansing or nourishing clay, fruit or oat mask can be applied once every two weeks to eliminate dead cells and promote regeneration, but be careful with the strongest fruit masks (those containing citrus juices, papaya, strawberry or tomato). In summer or after wind exposure, use herbal ice cubes (see page 32).

Hydrolats: chamomile, cornflower, lavender, orange blossom, rosemary, rosewater.

20s to 30s

See teens for cleansing, mask routine and herbal ice cubes. Begin to introduce recipes containing hydrating or toning ingredients, such as honey and cucumber milk (see page 54), rosewater, honey and lemon lotion (see page 111) and apple cologne (see page 104). Cosmetic vinegar (see page 46) is also good.

Essential oils: chamomile, geranium, lavender, niaouli, palmarosa, rosemary, rose otto, rosewood.

Carrier oils: hazelnut, olive, sweet almond.

Hydrolats: see teens.

30s to 40s

Use a gentle cleanser containing hydrating and balancing ingredients daily (see teens and 20s to 30s) and follow with a mild toner, such as rosewater and witchhazel cleanser (see page 62), apple cologne (see page 104) or rosewater astringent lotion (see page 106). Massage face and neck once a day with a suitable oil mix (see pages 34–44). Choose a cleansing and toning mask containing citrus juice (orange, grapefruit or lemon), dairy produce or honey, and use once a week.

Essential oils: see 20s to 30s.

Carrier oils: see 20s to 30s, plus apricot kernel, lime blossom, wheatgerm.

Hydrolats: see teens.

40s to 50s

See 30s to 40s for daily routine with cleanser, toner and massage. Once a week alternate a series of toning and nourishing masks and lotions. Avoid exfoliating ingredients such as papaya or tomato, which may now be too harsh for this type of skin, putting emphasis on nourishing recipes containing borage oil, evening primrose oil, wheatgerm or vitamin E oil.

Essential oils: see teens, substituting clary sage, cypress and frankincense for niaouli.

Carrier oils: see teens and 20s to 30s, plus macadamia nut.

Hydrolats: chamomile, clary sage, rosemary, rosewater, witchhazel.

50s+

see under ageing skin

dry skin

teens

Use daily a gentle cleanser, such as almond milk (see page 50). Avoid steaming, but compresses or herbal ice cubes (see pages 30–32) can be used at any time. Alternate hydrating blackcurrant and nourishing banana fruit masks, using one once or twice a week. An oat and lemon juice mask (see page 67) can be used once every two weeks to remove dead cells. The yoghurt and carrot juice mask (see page 76) is also an excellent way to nourish the skin and maintain a good pH. Experiment with the clay and cucumber recipe (see page 55), adding 2 tablespoons of olive or sweet almond oil. Massage face and neck once a day with a suitable oil mix (see pages 34–44).

Essential oils: chamomile, geranium, lavender, palmarosa, rosemary, rose otto, rosewood.

Carrier oils: olive, sweet almond.

Hydrolats: orange blossom, rosemary, rosewater.

20s to 30s

See teens. The honey and cucumber cleansing milk (see page 54) is another gentle cleanser which can be used daily.

Essential oils: see teens, plus frankincense, neroli.

Carrier oils: apricot kernel, macadamia nut, olive, wheatgerm.

Hydrolats: clary sage, rosemary, rosewater.

30s to 40s

See teens and 20s to 30s for daily cleansing, the clay and cucumber cleansing mask and advice on steaming, compresses, ice cubes and massage. Alternate nourishing, hydrating and toning masks containing avocado, banana, blackcurrant and grape as appropriate, once a week. A simple oat mask with 1 added teaspoon of lemon juice (see page 27) can be used occasionally to eliminate dead cells, tone and promote regeneration. The spirulina mask (see page 74) and the healing mask (see page 89) are also excellent for nourishing and revitalising the skin. Experiment with any recipe which combines ingredients that nourish (honey and cream) with those that tone (lemon and egg white).

Essential oils: see teens and 20s to 30s, omitting lavender.

Carrier oils: see 20s to 30s, plus borage.

Hydrolats: see 20s to 30s, plus chamomile, cornflower, witchhazel.

40s to 50s

see under ageing skin

50s+

see under ageing skin

oily skin

teens

Use daily a simple cleansing lotion, such as rosewater and lemon juice (see page 59) or a chamomile infusion (see page 30). That and steaming (see page 33) once a week may be all that is needed to prevent clogged pores, inflammation and fatty deposits under the skin. Once every one or two weeks apply a clay mask made with cucumber juice (see page 55) or a chamomile infusion, (see page 30) and no more than once a month try a clay mask, using orange or grapefruit juice, or a fruit mask containing raspberry or tomato. Cosmetic vinegar (see page 46) is also helpful. Massage face and neck once a day with a suitable oil mix (see pages 34–44).

Essential oils: cedarwood, chamomile, cypress, juniper, lavender, lemon, mandarin, patchouli, rosewood.

Carrier oils: calendula, hazelnut, hypericum, jojoba, olive, sweet almond.

Hydrolats: chamomile, lavender, orange blossom, rosewater.

20s to 30s

See teens. For deeper cleansing, use the pineapple (see page 65) or papaya exfoliators (see page 68) to remove blackheads and spots.

Essential oils, carrier oils and hydrolats: see teens.

30s to 40s

See teens and 20s to 30s.

Essential oils: see teens, plus niaouli and tea tree.

Carrier oils and hydrolats: see teens.

40s to 50s

Use daily a gentle cleanser, such as almond (see page 50) or honey and cucumber milk (see page 54), and continue massage. Steam once every two weeks (see page 33); compresses or ice cubes (see pages 30–32) can be used frequently. Try the clay and cucumber cleansing mask (see page 55), adding 1 tablespoon of borage oil. Use a nourishing banana or hydrating blackcurrant fruit mask once a week, plus an oat mask with added lemon juice (see page 27) every two or three weeks to promote regeneration. Experiment with toners and recipes using yoghurt, cream or honey.

Essential oils: chamomile, clary sage, cypress, frankincense, geranium, lavender, lemon, myrrh, rosemary, rose otto, rosewood.

Carrier oils: apricot kernel, macadamia nut, olive, wheatgerm.

Hydrolats: chamomile, clary sage, cornflower, orange blossom, rosemary, rosewater.

50s+

see under ageing skin

combination skin

teens

Steam (see page 33) once weekly to check oily areas, but use daily a gentle cleaner, such as almond milk (see page 50) or a chamomile infusion (see page 30). Once every one or two weeks apply a clay mask made with cucumber juice (see page 55) or chamomile infusion, and once a month a clay mask, using orange or grapefruit juice, or a raspberry or tomato fruit mask. Massage face and neck once a day with a suitable oil mix (see pages 34–44).

Essential oils: cedarwood, chamomile, cypress, lavender, lemon, mandarin, neroli, patchouli, rosewood, tea tree.

Carrier oils: calendula, hazelnut, hypericum, jojoba, olive, sweet almond.

Hydrolats: chamomile, lavender, orange blossom, rosewater.

20s to 30s

Using almond milk (see page 50), rosewater and lemon juice (see page 59) or clay milk (see page 58), cleanse the face daily. Steam once a week (see page 33) and apply a clay mask using carrot juice, not water (see pages 22–24), or try a yoghurt- or oat-based mask. Apply a clay and citrus-juice mask or fruit mask (see teens) every two or three weeks. Cosmetic vinegar (see page 46) is also useful.

Essential oils, carrier oils and hydrolats: see teens.

30s to 40s

For steaming, daily cleansing, massage, fruit masks and cosmetic vinegar, see 20s to 30s, minus the cleansing milk. Once a week apply a clay mask made with carrot juice, not water (see pages 22–24), or with geranium oil (see page 73), or a yoghurt- or oat-based mask. Consider regular use of a toning mask or lotion, such as barley and rosemary lotion (see page 108), fresh juice toner (see page 110), or yoghurt and blackcurrant mask (see page 99).

Essential oils, carrier oils and hydrolats: see teens.

40s to 50s

A combination skin tends to become dry now. For daily cleansing, massage and cosmetic vinegar, see 20s to 30s. For a once-weekly mask, see 30s to 40s. Every two or three weeks try an extra-nourishing clay mask, adding 2 tablespoons of chopped parsley to the basic mix (see page 23), or the spirulina vitalising mask (see page 74). For regular toning, see 30s to 40s.

Essential oils: see teens, substituting clary sage, frankincense, geranium, for mandarin.

Carrier oils: see teens, plus borage.

Hydrolats: see teens, plus clary sage.

50s+

see under ageing skin

ageing skin

30s to 40s

Constant nourishing and toning is essential for skin showing signs of premature ageing. Use daily an astringent and toning cleanser, such as rosewater and lemon juice (see page 59) or rosewater and witchhazel (see page 62). Twice a week, do a nourishing mask, such as the spirulina vitalising mask (see page 74), banana anti-ageing mask (see page 72), high nutrient and vitamin mask (see page 88) or almond and egg white mask (see page 81). If possible, apply daily a toner, such as fresh juice toner (see page 110) or cucumber and vinegar lotion (see page 107), or one of the toning and hydrating masks. Use cosmetic vinegar (see page 46) when washing your face or in the bath. Daily massage and the application of essential oils becomes an even more important part of the fight against dehydration (see pages 34–44).

Essential oils: cedarwood, chamomile, clary sage, cypress, frankincense, geranium, lavender, myrrh, palmarosa, rose otto, rosewood, sandalwood.

Carrier oils: apricot kernel, borage, evening primrose, hazelnut, hypericum, lime blossom, macadamia nut, olive, rosehip seed, wheatgerm.

Hydrolats: chamomile, clary sage, cornflower, orange blossom, rosewater.

40s to 50s

See 30s to 40s.

Essential oils, carrier oils and hydrolats: see 30s to 40s.

50s+

See 30s to 40s. The oil mixture for daily massage should be a prepared blend of 50ml rosehip seed and 50ml lime blossom as joint carriers (if unavailable, use hypericum or olive) plus 2ml clary sage, 1ml geranium, 1ml frankincense and 1ml sandalwood essential oils (see pages 34–44).

Essential oils, carrier oils and hydrolats: see 30s to 40s.

sensitive skin

teens

Use a chamomile infusion (see page 30) daily as a face wash, followed by the traditional almond milk (see page 50) or honey and cucumber cleansing milk (see page 54). The hydrolats listed below can be used as often as you like (see also page 45). Make an oil mix, using olive oil as the carrier with a blend of lavender, rosewood and tea tree, and massage the face and neck once a day (see pages 34–44). Be careful with any treatment that may be too harsh for a sensitive skin, such as masks containing strawberry, tomato or papaya, but once every two weeks use an oat and lemon juice mask, substituting an infusion of chamomile for the witchhazel (see page 67). Use cosmetic vinegar (see page 46) when washing your face or in the bath.

Essential oils: cedarwood, chamomile, cypress, lavender, lemon, rosewood, tea tree.

Carrier oils: calendula, hazelnut, olive, sweet almond.

Hydrolats: chamomile, cornflower, lavender, orange blossom, rosewater.

20s to 30s

See teens. Alternate the mask you apply once every two weeks, using the oat and lemon juice mask with a chamomile infusion (see page 67, VARIATION), light nourishing masks such as yoghurt and carrot juice (see page 76), or the toning yoghurt and blackcurrant (see page 99).

Essential oils: see teens, plus frankincense.

Carrier oils: see teens.

Hydrolats: see teens.

30s to 40s

See teens, adding the alternative masks under 20s to 30s. An astringent and toning cleanser such as rosewater and lemon juice (see page 59) can also be used every day.

Essential oils: see teens, plus frankincense.

Carrier oils: see teens, plus borage or evening primrose.

Hydrolats: see teens.

40s to 50s

see under ageing skin

50s+

see under ageing skin

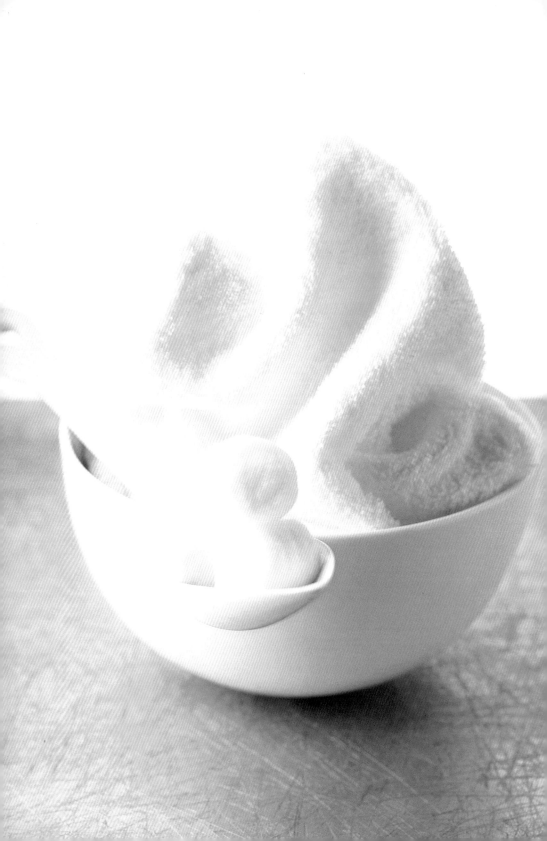

basic
techniques

masks and lotions

The masks and lotions in this book offer all the basic tools you need for short- and long-term natural skin care. Sourcing your skin products from simple, seasonal, raw ingredients means that you have immediate and direct access to a complex mixture of natural substances far more beneficial to your skin than the synthetic counterparts used in many of today's commercial cosmetics. And, because these recipes are so inexpensive and simple to make, you have the opportunity to build a skin-care programme that responds week by week, season by season, to the current state of your skin, whatever your environment.

clay

Clay is a very versatile ingredient in skin care. As a deep cleanser, it detoxifies by drawing impurities out from beneath the epidermis. As a nourisher, it contributes trace elements important to the maintenance of healthy skin. As a toner, its astringent action is best associated with ingredients such as lemon juice or hydrolats (see page 45). Therapeutically, clay is also antiseptic, anti-inflammatory and analgesic.

TYPES OF CLAY

A sediment formed by the slow erosion of granite, clay contains various minerals, such as iron oxide, salts, calcium and other trace elements in varying proportions, which alter its colour and therapeutic qualities. Three kinds are commonly available for cosmetic purposes.

White clay (or kaolin) is rich in silica and magnesium. This clay is neutral and not too drying, and it is effective in absorbing impurities and putting valuable minerals back into the skin. It is suitable for all types of skin (and especially those with dry skin) as a mask or lotion. Green clay (or montmorillonite) brings more mineral and trace elements to the skin, being rich in silica, manganese, potassium, aluminium and iron oxide, but it is also more drying. Its powerful action is most suitable for problem skin conditions, including acne, seborrhoea, eczema or damaged skin. Red clay (also montmorillonite, or sometimes illite or attapulgite) has properties and indications similar to those of green clay. Its red colour is due to a high concentration of iron oxide.

Cosmetic clay is available in three forms apart from the ready-made masks sold at greatly inflated prices. You may find it in an enter-prising supermarket but there are a number of specialist suppliers (see page 128). Buy it in powder form if you can. This is easy to use, absorbing water or any other liquid rapidly and mixing well with other solid ingredients, such as blue-green algae (also called spirulina), chopped herbs or puréed fruit or vegetables. Clay sold in small lumps takes slightly longer to mix, unless you powder it yourself first in a food processor, blender or coffee grinder. Finally, clay is also sold as a paste, ready to use. Although this is clearly time-saving, it does limit the sort of mask you can make because some recipes require that other ingredients are added to the clay before the liquid. It is also relatively more expensive.

MAKING A CLAY MASK

The method of making a basic clay mask is very simple. The required amount of clay (usually 2–3 tablespoons) is just covered with still min-eral water (say, by 5mm) and left to rest for a minimum of 30 minutes without stirring. Evian water or some other bottled water which is low on minerals is recommended; do not use tap water or any water which contains chlorine. It is important not to stir until after the resting period (when all the water has been absorbed) because premature stirring affects the consistency of the mask, making it sticky and lumpy and therefore more difficult to apply.

Once the resting period is over, the ingredients are stirred thoroughly to mix well. To be ready to use, the mixture must have the consistency of a thick paste which can be applied with ease. If it is too liquid, it will not adhere; if it is too thick, it will not penetrate deeply into the skin. It is easy enough to add a small amount of clay to a mix which is too thin, but adding more water to a paste which is too thick requires great care: add very gradually, stirring all the time.

If other ingredients are to be added to the clay, it is preferable to do so at this stage, but any oil or blend of oils (see page 37) are best added to the dry clay. Some of the recipes in this book substitute fruit or vegetable juices or hydrolats for still bottled water. The same rules on resting and stirring apply. Clay powder (or potato flour) is also used as a thickening agent in some lighter masks. No resting time is necessary in most cases – follow the recipe instructions. To be effective, a clay mask is best applied at least once or twice a week. See pages 27–29 for how to make the most of a clay mask, including application and removal.

fruit

Many of the fruits we eat everyday make excellent masks that have a revitalising, nourishing and often astringent action on the skin. It is the variety of acids they contain (including malic, glycolic, citric, salicylic and tartric acid) and their high vitamin and mineral content that bring these benefits.

Indeed, fruit acids are now extracted (alpha-hydroxy acids) or chemically synthesised (beta-hydroxy acids) commercially and used by cosmetic surgeons as chemical peeling agents at high concentrations for those prepared to suffer pain and risk burns, allergic reactions and hypersensitisation to the sun in pursuit of a more youthful appearance.

Fortunately, the natural ingredients in simple fruit masks – in which the crushed flesh or juice of fresh fruits is applied directly to the skin – have a milder action, acting in synergy without dangerous side effects. All the fruit masks in this book can be applied frequently and are beneficial in many ways for a variety of skin types, especially for those with dry or ageing skin.

Their gentle peeling action removes dead skin, excess fatty deposits and blackheads from the epidermis and eliminates freckles and excess pigmentation, making the skin appear whiter, as well as erasing faint lines and wrinkles of expression. By increasing the acidity on the surface of the skin, they also inhibit the growth of bacteria, help regulate the secretion of sebum, unclog and close pores and tone and hydrate the skin. In addition they contribute small amounts of trace elements and minerals essential for healthy skin, such as potassium, zinc and selenium.

However, there is one warning note to sound for anyone who has sensitive skin or is potentially allergic. It is not wise to use highly acidic fruit masks (such as tomatoes) more than once a week. It might also be sensible to test on a small portion of the skin on the inside arm for possible allergic reactions. Apply a small amount directly to the skin, leave for 2–3 minutes, remove with a cottonwool ball, wait a further 10 minutes and then check for any redness where the mask was applied.

USING FRUIT FOR MASKS AND LOTIONS

The best fruits to use for cleansing, toning and nourishing are apple, apricot, avocado, banana, blackcurrant, cherry, grape, grapefruit, lemon, melon, orange, raspberry, papaya, pineapple and tomato. Use the freshest fruit you can find, preferably organically grown, and, if a recipe requires fruit juices, make them yourself whenever possible, again using fresh ingredients. Cartoned fresh carrot and grape juice are acceptable but avoid long-life, UHT and canned products.

Most fruit masks and lotions are extremely easy to make either by hand or using a food processor or liquidiser/blender. The fruit is crushed to a purée or its juice is extracted, and the resulting product is simply and speedily mixed with other natural ingredients, such as dairy products, honey, eggs, hydrolats (see page 45) or oils (see pages 34–41). If the consistency of a purée needs a bulking agent to make a mask that can be easily applied, a small amount of clay powder, oatmeal, potato flour or live organic yoghurt is often added without compromising its benefits. Juices from fruits such as grapefruit, lemon, orange, grape or tomato are also mixed with larger amounts of clay or with stiffly beaten egg white to create an effective mask, or applied directly to the skin as a lotion either alone or in association with other natural ingredients, using cottonwool balls. See pages 27–29 for how to make the most of masks and lotions.

vegetables

Masks based on fresh vegetable ingredients have an anti-inflammatory action, making them a must for sensitive, damaged or inflamed skin. In addition to their cooling properties, they promote healing by giving to the damaged epidermis large amounts of vitamin A, plus important minerals and trace elements. This means that vegetable masks are most valuable at times of crisis – for sudden outbreaks of acne or eczema, or for sunburn or allergic reactions to food or medical drugs – although they are good for cleansing and nourishing too.

USING VEGETABLES FOR MASKS AND LOTIONS

The most valuable vegetables for skin care are cabbage, carrot, cucumber, lettuce, potato and watercress. The herb parsley is also beneficial. Always use the freshest possible ingredients, organically grown if available, and make your own juice whenever possible.

For more general skin care, the options are very straightforward. Cucumber (grated or juiced) can be added to clay for a number of effective masks, and cucumber or carrot juice can be applied directly to the skin in association with other ingredients as a lotion. Fresh parsley or watercress can simply be chopped and added to a clay mask or to live organic yoghurt or double cream. And with very little more effort the green vegetables – lettuce, watercress or cabbage – can be puréed and then thickened with clay or oatmeal to apply as a mask. Alternatively, the cooked and cooled leaves of lettuce or cabbage can be applied directly to the skin, and the cooking water used as a gentle lotion. Potato flour (or clay) is also used as a bulking agent in some lighter masks. See pages 27–29 for how to make the most of masks and lotions.

other ingredients

Barley In the recipes in this book only barley water is used, in a lotion, but cooked barley can be processed into a paste and used as a mask.
Dairy Full-cream milk and live organic yoghurt are used to balance and cleanse, whereas cream (and it must be thick double cream) adds

nourishment. Thickener is essential in any dairy-based mask. See eggs for advice on storage.

Eggs Yolks are added to masks to make them more nourishing and to thicken; stiffly beaten whites make a mask more astringent and easier to spread and adhere. Masks containing egg must be used quickly, although they can be stored for 6 hours in a refrigerator.

Honey Usually added to other substances such as clay, eggs, fruit or yoghurt, honey enhances the nourishing qualities of a mask or a lotion. It also acts as a thickening and 'adhesive' agent.

Oats Fine oatmeal, bran or coarser porridge oats can be used cooked or raw as the basis of a mask. Cooked in water and cooled, they can be used as a mask. Uncooked, they can be bound with water (sometimes with 1 teaspoon of lemon juice) or with milk or yoghurt; in this state they are often extremely absorbent. Oatmeal is also an excellent thickener.

Pollen A teaspoon of powdered or ground pollen enriches any mask and is very useful for ageing or damaged skin. Add a little more liquid – fruit juice, water or hydrolat – as the recipe dictates.

Royal jelly Because of its creamy consistency, royal jelly can be added to a mask without further adjustment just before it is applied to the skin.

IMPORTANT: BEFORE YOU MAKE A MASK
Most metals oxidise in contact with clay, fruit or vegetable juices so avoid using metal mixing bowls or containers. Similarly, do not use a metal spoon or spatula for stirring, although the stainless-steel blades of a processor or liquidiser are fine. Make sure that all equipment is absolutely clean. If in doubt, pour boiling water over it to sterilise. The quantities indicated for some of the recipes may vary according to the quality of the ingredients or the weather. In dry, hot weather, for example, you may need to add more liquid. It is assumed that you are using a small blender or processor; there will inevitably be more wastage on family models and you may have to double quantities. Warm water may be used in a mask, but never heat a preparation. And don't be tempted to save time by making large quantities. Masks are best made just before they are used, although the recipes specify shelf-life.

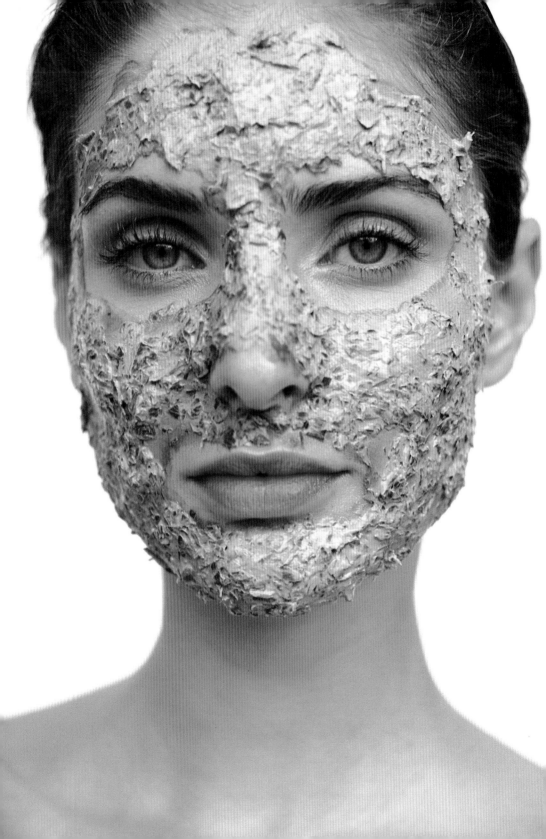

applying masks and lotions

The following sequence sets out the ideal way to use a natural mask or lotion. Sadly, many of us today lead such busy lives that we find it difficult to devote so much time to ourselves. Aim to find that time perhaps once a week and, when that is not possible, skip step 4 and maybe combine steps 2 and 3.

1 Find yourself a quiet, calm time and place. When you allow yourself the space to slow down and enjoy the simple processes of preparing, applying and removing a mask, you are likely to be more centred, and that means more receptive and responsive.

2 Put on a towelling band and remove any makeup. Then carefully clean the skin with cottonwool balls and still bottled water, a herbal infusion (see page 30), using chamomile, rosemary or lavender flowers, a hydrolat (see page 45) or one of the simpler cleansing recipes (see pages 50 and 59).

3 Relax your facial muscles in any way that suits you. It might be by using massage or by making hideous faces at yourself in the mirror.

4 Steam your face gently (1–2 minutes over a bowl of hot water) or apply a hot compress for 2 minutes (see pages 32 and 33). Both techniques open the pores so that the mask can penetrate more deeply.

5 Apply the mask evenly, avoiding the area around the eyes (unless, of course, it is an eye mask) and using your fingers or cottonwool balls as appropriate. Fruit or egg masks often have a very liquid consistency. It may be easier to apply a second layer after a few minutes, once the first layer has dried a little.

6 Try not to talk, laugh or even move any facial muscle until it is time to gently remove the mask.

7 Remove the mask slowly and carefully. Work from the forehead downwards, making sure that none of the material removed comes into contact with the eyes, and avoid dragging the skin. Light fruit masks can be removed simply with cottonwool balls. With clay masks, you need to rinse the face first to soften the clay.

8 Where appropriate, spray or apply a hydrolat to close the pores and tone the skin. See the recipes and the listings on pages 14–19 for guidance.

herbal infusions

Fresh and dried herbs have been used to make infusions with medical properties, applied externally or used with compresses, for thousands of years. The list below outlines the properties and benefits of the principle herbs recommended for use in herbal infusions. Several have cleansing and toning qualities which make them useful in any long-term natural skin-care programme; all are suitable for any type of skin.

Calendula (marigold flower) Antiseptic, anti-fungal, anti-inflammatory, healing. Use alone or in a half-and-half mix with lavender or chamomile.

Chamomile flower Best anti-inflammatory for a frequently irritated skin, anti-fungal, soothing, cleansing. The infusion is especially recommended for the fragile skin around the eyes.

Elder flower Astringent, anti-inflammatory, cleansing, toning.

Lavender flower Anti-inflammatory, soothing, cleansing. Lavender is slightly drying.

Lime flower Similar to chamomile, very calming. Its mildly toning, anti-inflammatory effect is good for ageing skin.

Mallow Gentle anti-inflammatory, soothing, calming.

Mint Good toner.

Rosemary Antiseptic, toning and vitalising; improves blood circulation in the capillaries. Use rosemary alone or in a half-and-half mix with yarrow for a more astringent effect.

Thyme Strong anti-bacterial effect: useful as a skin wash for acne or infected eczema. Use alone or in equal parts with chamomile and/or calendula to soothe and heal.

Yarrow Good toner, astringent, antiseptic for ageing or damaged skin.

TO MAKE A SIMPLE INFUSION

Use 1 generous tablespoon of dried chopped herbs to 250ml (8¾fl.oz) of boiling water. Placing the herbs in an average-sized mug and filling it to the brim will do the trick. Leave to infuse for 10 minutes, strain, reserve the liquid and leave to cool before using. Apply with cotton-wool balls or in a mister and leave to dry naturally.

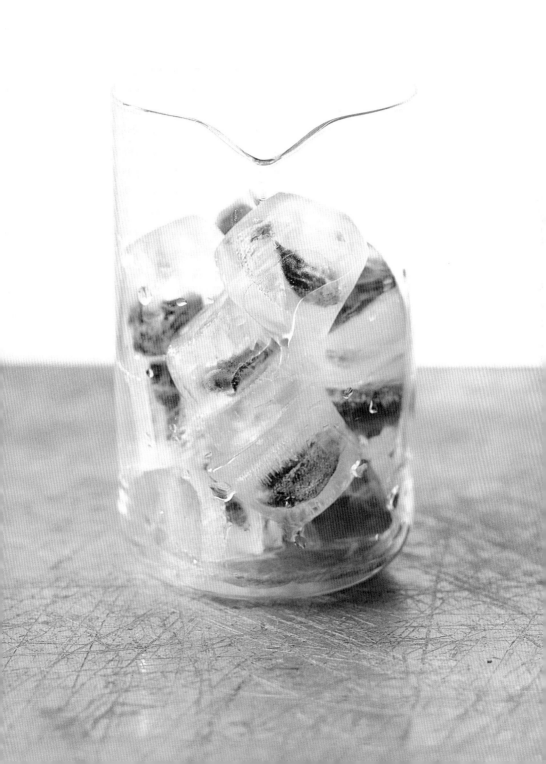

INFUSIONS FOR ICE CUBES

An infusion has a shelf life of about 12 hours so don't be tempted to bottle large quantities. However, you can freeze a strained and cooled infusion in an ice-cube tray and keep it in the freezer compartment of your refrigerator for up to 1 month or 3 months in a freezer. The recommended infusions for ice cubes are: chamomile, lavender, lime flower and rosemary. The hydrolats listed on page 45 can also be diluted to make ice cubes. Allow 1 tablespoon of hydrolat per 100ml (3½fl.oz) of still bottled water.

To use, simply rub a cube directly on your face, neck and arms for a deliciously cooling and hydrating effect. It also has a toning action, of course, because it quickens the blood circulation in the cap-illaries of the dermis.

INFUSIONS FOR COMPRESSES

Compresses also tone the skin – improving blood circulation, hydrating and closing the pores – as well as calming inflammation. Especially good for dry, ageing or damaged skin, they can be used occasionally on any skin type.

Ideally you need two large bowls, but you may be able to impro-vise with one bowl and a bathroom basin. You also need two small face towels or flannels. Place 1 generous tablespoon of any of the dried herbs listed on page 30 and 1 tablespoon of lemon juice in one of the bowls, and pour on 3 mugs of boiling water. Leave to infuse for 15 minutes. Into the second bowl pour about 1 litre (2 pints) of cold water and 1 tablespoon of cider vinegar. Add a few ice cubes to chill.

Immerse one of the towels (or flannels) in the hot infusion and squeeeze out the excess water before laying the towel on the face and leaving it for about 1 minute. Take care: it will be hot at first. Remove the first towel and quickly dip the other towel into the cold water bowl. Apply to the face in the same way, again leaving for 1 minute. Repeat this procedure twice, alternating hot and cold compresses. It is important to finish with a cold compress to close the pores. Finish by dabbing on rosewater hydrolat (see page 45) and leaving to dry naturally.

steaming

One traditional and very simple way to deep clean the skin is to steam your face for a few minutes from time to time. Steaming removes dirt and pollution very efficiently from the skin, but it removes important natural oils as well. So, although the technique brings excellent results on an oily skin or for anyone suffering from acne, most skin types must bear in mind that in the long term it has a drying effect.

Steaming should therefore be used very occasionally on a dry or ageing skin (once in a month is the maximum) and never for more than 2–3 minutes. On a oily skin, it can be done once or twice every seven days, and for 6–8 minutes at a time. For a combination skin, 2–3 minutes once a week is the recommended maximum. A normal skin will benefit from an occasional steaming (every two weeks), as long as the exposure to steam is not prolonged (5 minutes maximum). It is not recommended for extremely sensitive skins, for anyone suffering from severe inflammation, infection or sunburn, from rosacea, or for those who have many small blood vessels visible on the surface of the skin. However, these conditions respond very well to the regular application of clay masks (see the Cleansing recipes for dry or ageing skin).

TO STEAM

All you need, of course, is a large bowl containing about 1 litre (2 pints) of boiling water and a medium-sized towel. Sit before the bowl, cover your head with the towel and keep your face in the steam for the recommended time. Then pat your face dry with cottonwool balls or a towel and tone with rosewater hydrolat (see page 45), leaving the skin to dry naturally.

The benefits of steaming can be enhanced by adding 2 drops of chamomile, geranium, lavender, rose otto or tea tree essential oil (see pages 34 and 40–41) to the boiling water. After drying, apply a thin film of the same oil to the skin, diluted in a calendula carrier (see pages 34–37).

aromatherapy

Essential oils are an excellent and safe alternative to cosmetic and conventional medical treatment of the skin. I have been using them for years with great success to treat the most difficult cases of eczema and rosacea, but they are also irreplaceable for daily skin care. For confirmation, you only have to look at the ingredients list of most cosmetic products. In this book you will find essential and carrier oils used in the recipe sections – to cleanse, to nourish and to tone – for steaming (see page 33), for massage (see page 42–44) and for the treatment of common skin conditions (see pages 114–125).

ESSENTIAL OILS

Found in the roots, leaves, stems or flowers of aromatic plants, in the bark of trees such as pine, fir and cinnamon, and in the peel of some citrus fruits, essential oils are a complex mixture of up to 250 chemicals. These fragrant substances, synthesised in plants by the energy of the sun, are mostly extracted by the ancient process of steam distillation. A few, for example the citrus oils, are obtained by cold expression; rose absolute is derived by chemical extraction and is inferior to the recommended form, rose otto.

They have such a complex chemistry that it remains impossible to know exactly how they work. But, scientific analysis in the late twentieth century classified the families of molecules commonly found in essential oils and that has helped to explain some of the therapeutic effects consistently observed in aromatherapy, such as the destruction or inhibition of viruses and bacteria, anti-inflammatory action and hormone regulation.

CARRIER OILS

Because of their powerful effects, essential oils are only very rarely used undiluted directly on the skin (see Safety on page 36). Much gentler vegetable oils are used to dilute the essential oils used for massage and are known in consequence as carrier oils. Although any vegetable oil could be used, cold-pressed oils obtained from nuts or seeds are preferred for their therapeutic properties and because they can act in synergy with specific essential oils for additional benefits – a case of two plus two making five. Cold-pressed oils are expensive, but they are much more beneficial than the cheaper, industrially extracted oils, containing varying but larger quantities of valuable vitamins, trace elements and fatty acids. They are also economical in use.

CHOOSING CARRIER OILS

The first step in choosing oils for massage or to treat common skin problems is to select a carrier (or carriers). A chart listing the characteristics of all the major carrier oils appears on pages 38–39. The programmes in Caring for your skin give the appropriate carrier oils for each skin type and every age group (see pages 14–19). Sweet almond and olive oil will suit any kind of skin, and can serve either as a single carrier or as the larger part of a blend of carriers.

It is very important to choose the right carrier oil: each has its own specific action, but it can also diffuse or enhance the therapeutic qualities of the essential oils it carries. When selecting a carrier oil for massage, try one oil at a time. If it feels right, it probably is – so long as you've assessed your skin type and its condition correctly (see page 12). You may sometimes need to blend two, possibly three, carriers which suit your skin type, age group and skin condition, but most of the time only one is needed. Blends of two or three carrier oils are used for their therapeutic effects or for economy.

Therapeutically, for example, calendula oil works well in synergy with hypericum oil for very oily, damaged or inflamed skin. And for reasons of economy, no more than 10–15 per cent of jojoba or macadamia nut carrier oils, or of borage, evening primrose, rosehip seed or vitamin E supplementary oils, are usually blended with a cheaper carrier such as apricot kernel, olive or sweet almond oil.

Quality olive, sweet almond and wheatgerm oils are easily available, while the others can be ordered from reputable specialists (see page 126).

CHOOSING ESSENTIAL OILS

You can use a blend of up to four essential oils in the single or blended carrier oils used for massage or to treat common skin conditions. A chart listing all the essential oils recommended and their main benefits appears on pages 40–41. The programmes for lifelong skin care in Caring for your skin give the appropriate essential oils for each skin type and age group (see pages 14–19).

The principle oil for any blend of essential oils for massage must satisfy your main objective: for example, to hydrate the skin or to regulate excessive sebum. You may then choose smaller amounts of one or two other oils that will enhance and complement the action of your principal oil. Finally, one more oil can be selected either as a balancer – to counteract any possible over-action of the other oils – or to treat some other symptom of your skin. The selected essential oils are measured and blended in a separate container before being added in the required quantity to your carrier: the total amount of essential oil should never be more than 3.5 per cent of the resulting preparation. See opposite for detailed instructions on blending oils.

SAFETY PRECAUTIONS

Most essential oils are safe for home use if they are used correctly. However, they are best avoided during the early months of pregnancy. After the third or fourth month, chamomile, geranium, lavender, neroli, patchouli, rose otto, rosewood and sandalwood are recommended. Cedarwood, clary sage, juniper, myrrh and rosemary should be avoided throughout pregnancy. Essential oils are concentrated substances so keep them out of children's reach; in particular, never leave a bottle without a fixed dropper where a child could drink the contents.

Unless personally advised by an expert, and with the few following exceptions, never apply neat essential oil to the skin. It must be diluted in a carrier oil first. But lavender can be used neat on burns, tea tree on athlete's foot, and rose otto or sandalwood as a perfume. Avoid immediate exposure to strong sunlight or ultraviolet light after using mandarin. It is slightly phototoxic, which means it can cause skin discoloration, so be careful how you use it in summertime. Juniper should always be used sparingly as it can sometimes cause mild skin irritation.

Most essential oils, even when diluted, will cause stinging if they get into the eyes. If you splash neat essential oil into your eyes, flush them immediately with milk or with a carrier or vegetable oil, and, if the stinging and irritation continues, seek medical assistance quickly. If the essential oil is diluted, flush immediately with a carrier oil.

BLENDING OILS

While you are experimenting with various mixes, it is best to make enough for just one day's massage. One tablespoon (that's 10ml) of carrier oil and 10 drops of essential oil in total are all you need. Consult the recommendations for your skin type and age on pages 14–19 and the charts on pages 38–41 to select the appropriate carrier and essential oils. To keep it simple at first, choose a single carrier and two essential oils (5 drops of each).

Once you are satisfied with a particular blend, it makes sense to prepare a larger amount – these oils have a shelf life of about three months. For the contents of a 30ml bottle of carrier oil(s), you will need an essential-oil blend totalling 30 drops; for a 50ml bottle of carrier oil(s), the essential oils will total 50 drops. (Viscosities vary but on average 1ml = 40 drops of essential oil.)

To blend oils in quantity, you need two brown glass bottles – light degrades the benefits of essential oils. You will find them in aromatherapy shops and many local pharmacies (see page 126 for mail-order). One must be large enough to hold your assembled preparation, but the other can be very small. This one will be used to blend your essential oils before they are added to the carrier(s) and it needs a removable dropper/top.

Begin by pouring the required amount of carrier oil(s) into the large bottle. Then combine the essential oils in the small bottle, close (using the dropper/top) and shake well. Finally add the essential oils to the carrier bottle, close and shake again to blend. Your oil mix is now ready to use.

carrier oils

	normal skin	dry skin	oily skin	combination skin	ageing skin	sensitive skin
apricot kernel	•••	•••••	•	••••	•••••	•••
calendula	•••	•	•••••	•••	••	•••••
hazelnut	••••	••	••••	••••	•••	•••
hypericum	•••	••	••••	•••	•••	••••
jojoba	•	•••	••••	•••	•	•••
lime blossom	••	•••	•	•••	•••••	•••••
macadamia nut	•	•••	••••	•••	•••	••
olive	•••••	•••••	•••••	•••••	•••••	••••
sweet almond	•••••	••••	•••	•••••	••••	••••
wheatgerm	••	•••••	•	•••	•••••	•••
borage or evening primrose	••	•••	•	•	•••••	•••••
rosehip seed	••	•••••	○	••	•••••	•••••
vitamin e	••	•••••	•	••	•••••	••••

○ = no potency   • = low potency   ••••• = high potency

damaged skin	anti-inflammatory	fungicidal	healing scars	nourishing	drying	regulating
•••••	•••	•	•••	••••	○	•••
•••••	•••••	••••	•••••	••	••••	•••
••••	••••	•	•••	••••	••	•••
•••	•••••	•	•••	•	••	••
•	•	•	•	•••	○	••••
•	••	•	•	•	○	•••
••	○	○	○	•••	○	••••
•••	••••	•	•••	••••	○	•••••
••••	••	•	••	•••	○	•••
••••	••	○	••••	•••	○	•••
••••	••	○	••••	•••	○	••••
•••••	•••	••	•••••	•••••	○	•••
•••••	••	○	•••••	•••••	○	•••

This table and that on pages 40–41 represent a broad evaluation based on practical experience. Supplementary oils are listed in italic and can be added in small quantities to carrier oils (see page 35).

essential oils

	normal skin	dry skin	oily skin	combination skin	ageing skin	sensitive skin	damaged skin	toxicity in pregnancy	anti-inflamme
cedarwood	••	•	••	••	••	o	•••••	•••	o
*chamomile *german*	••	•	•••	•••	•••	•••••	•••	•	•••••
*chamomile *roman*	••	•	•••	•••	•••	•••••	•••	•	•••
clary sage	••	•••	••	••	•••••	•••	•	•••••	•
cypress	••	•	•••••	••	••••	••	•••••	o	o
frankincense	••	••••	••	••	••••	••	•••••	o	•••
geranium	•••	•••••	•	•	•••	•••	•••	o	•••
juniper	•	•	•••	••	•	o	••	•••	•••
lavender	•••	••	•••••	••••	•••	••••	•••••	o	•••
lemon	••	••	••••	•••	••••	•	••••	o	••
mandarin	••	•	•••••	•••	•••	••••	••	o	•
myrrh	••	•••	•••	••	•••	•	••••	o	•••
neroli	•••	••••	•	••	••	•••	•••	o	•••
niaouli	•••	•••	•••	•••	•	•	••	••	•••
palmarosa	•••	•••	••	•••	•••	••	•••	o	••••
patchouli	••	••	•••	•••	•••	o	•••	o	•••
rose otto	•••	•••	••	••	•••••	•••	•••	••	•••
rosewood	•••	•••	•••	•••	•••	••••	•••	o	•••
rosemary	•••	•••	•••	•••	••••	••	•••••	•••••	•••
sandalwood	•••	•••	••	•••	••	•••	••	o	•
tea tree	•••	••	•••	•••	••	•••	•••	o	•••

o = no potency   • = low potency   ••••• = high potency

antibacterial	fungicidal	anti-viral	hydrating	regulating/balancing	calming	stimulating	healing scars	astringent	anti-allergic
○	○	○	○	●●	●	●	●●●●	●●	○
●●●	●●	○	○	●	●●●●●	○	●	○	●●
●●●	●●	○	○	●	●●●●	○	○	○	●
●	○	○	●●	●●●●	●●●●	○	○	●	○
●●●	●●●	○	○	●●●●	●●●	●	●●●●	●●●●	○
○	○	○	○	●●●	●●●	●	●●●●	●●	○
●●●	●●●	●	●●●●	●●●●	●●●	●	●	●	●
●●●●	●	○	○	○	●	●●	●●●	●●●	○
●●	●	●	○	●●●	●●●	○	●●●●	○	●●●
●●●●	●●●	●●●●	●	●●	○	●●●	●●	●●●●●	○
●	●	○	●	●●●	●●●●●	○	○	●●	○
●●●	●●	●●	●	●●●	●●	●	●●●●	●	○
●●●	●●	●	●	●●●	●●	●	●●●	○	○
●●●●	●●●	●●●●	●	●●	●	○	○	●	●
●●●	●●●	●●	●●	●●	●●	●	●●	●	●
●●●	●	○	●	●●	●	●●	●	●●	○
●●	○	○	●●	●●●	●	●●●	●	●●	●
●●●	●●●	●●●	●	●●	●●●	●●	○	●	●
●●	●●●	●●	●	●●●	○	●●●	●●	●●	○
●	○	○	●	●●●	●●	●●	○	●●	○
●●●●●	●●●●	●●●●	●	●	●	●●	○	○	○

*Use either where chamomile is specified. German chamomile is more concentrated.

MASSAGE TECHNIQUE

Regular massage with an appropriate blend of carrier and essential oils is an essential part of any good skin maintenance programme. An effective way to tone and generally improve the condition of any type of skin, it works by relaxing all the small muscles of the face, improving the circulation, breaking down fatty deposits in the lower levels of the skin and releasing toxins. Remember to make good use of it in association with masks and lotions as recommended for your skin type or condition (see pages 14–19 and 114–125). The sequence which follows repeats several simple techniques.

Technique 1 Use the tips of the index, middle and ring finger together to exert a deep, local pressure in a tiny circular movement. You should be able to feel the skin rubbing against the small muscles of the face. Lift the fingers and reposition them to travel across the skin.

Technique 2 Use the flat pads of the index, middle and ring fingers together or simply the thumb to travel across the skin – either in a slow, spiralling action or by simply sliding upwards, downwards or outwards. For the most part keep the remainder of your hand resting lightly on the face.

Pinching Use your index finger and thumb lightly but with enough strength to stimulate the circulation and cause a slight change of skin colour. Beware of bruising – pinch lightly on the eyebrows and upper face, more heavily along the jaw.

FACIAL MASSAGE SEQUENCE

Make sure you are sitting comfortably with everything you need at hand: towelling and/or elastic bands to secure your hair away from your face, a wet flannel or cloth to dampen your skin so that the oils emulsify and penetrate more easily, and a little massage oil poured onto a plate.

Warm-up Starting on either side of the nose, pinch along each eyebrow and as far as possible along the temples towards the tops of the ears. Then pinch from the chin, working slowly along the jawline and up to the base of the ears. Do this three times.

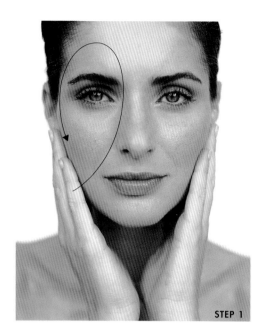

STEP 1

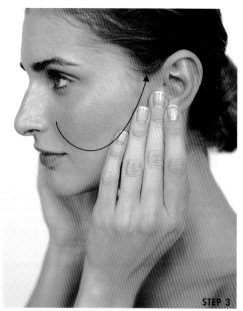

STEP 3

1   Dip the pads of your fingers into the oil and rub your palms together to spread it evenly. Place your fingertips on your jawbone and with light pressure make a large sweeping circle from the jawline up either side of the nose to the centre of the forehead, out along the hairline and then down the temples to meet at the jawbone. This gently stimulates the energy and spreads the oil.

2   With the tips of all three fingers and the local pressure of technique 1, start at the chin and travel along the jawline and then up from the angles of the jaw to the temples. Do this three times.

3   Using the pads of the three fingers and the small spiralling movement of technique 2, begin on each side of the nose, close to the base of the nostrils, moving first under the cheekbones and then up towards the tops of the ears.

4   Placing the tips of the middle fingers at the inner corners of the eyes, slide your fingers upwards, pushing against the orbital bone, and then outwards, just above the eyebrows, towards the ears.

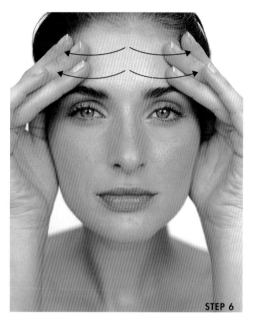

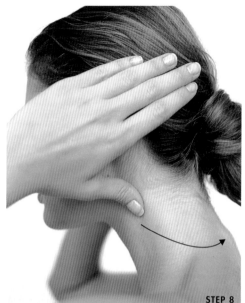

STEP 6

STEP 8

5 Use the pads of all three fingers and the spiralling movement of technique 2 to massage the forehead, starting just above the top of the nose and moving up towards the hairline and then outwards along it until you reach the temples.

6 Using technique 2, position the pads of all three fingers at the base of the central frown line, just above the top of the nose, and slide them toward the temples. Do this three times.

7 Massage your scalp firmly, as if you were shampooing your hair. Begin at the temples and work downwards, behind the ears and towards the base of the skull.

8 Resting your palms on your ears so that the thumbs point downwards, massage from your throat to the nape of the neck in a broad, spiralling version of technique 2. Do this three times.

9 Place one hand, palm down, each side of your nose. Your fingertips should rest slightly above your eyebrows. With firm, even pressure, slide your hands outwards towards the ears. Do three times.

10 Bring the sequence to an end by repeating the sweeping movement described in step 1.

hydrolats

Also known as hydrosols or floral waters (*not* flower waters), hydrolats are a by-product of steam distillation, created while extracting essential oil. They have properties similar to their related essential oils, although in a less concentrated form, but they are enriched with various water-soluble active ingredients. Their gentleness makes them an excellent way to tone, hydrate and rebalance the pH of the skin so they are frequently recommended as a cleanser/toner after cleansing or nourishing masks. Most also have a bactericidal, anti-viral action and can disinfect sensitive or damaged skin less harshly than detergents or alcohol-based lotions. All are available from specialist shops or by mail order (see page 126).

USING HYDROLATS

Hydrolats can be applied to the face twice daily. Use cottonwool or decant into a spray bottle, but take care to avoid the eyes (see corn-flower). Leave to dry naturally. Hydrolats can also be added to a bath as a general skin tonic (use 3 tablespoons) and are sometimes substituted for water when preparing clay masks (see page 23).

Chamomile Suitable for all skin types; very gentle anti-inflammatory, soothing and cleansing, good for over-exposure to sun and wind.

Clary sage Suitable for dry and ageing skin; for skin problems associated with fluctuating hormone levels and menopause.

Cornflower See chamomile. Often used around the eyes because, unlike most hydrolats, it does not burn in contact with them.

Lavender Suitable for all skin types, but slightly drying; cooling, anti-inflammatory, good for sun- or wind-burn and as hair tonic.

Orange blossom Suitable for all skin types, especially dry or sensitive skin; anti-inflammatory, good for rosacea.

Rosemary Excellent for balancing and toning all skin types and for hair; stimulates circulation.

Rosewater Suitable for all skin types, especially ageing; balancing, tonic, astringent.

Witchhazel Suitable for all skin types; mildly astringent, toning.

cosmetic vinegar

The use of vinegar with a variety of plants or essential oils for cosmetic purposes can be traced back to the Romans and was again fashionable during the nineteenth century as *vinaigre de toilette*.

Vinegar has a tonic action which promotes blood circulation in the small capillaries that irrigate the skin. It is also antiseptic, preventing the proliferation of bacteria, viruses or yeast that trigger infection. It can dissolve excessive fatty deposits at the surface of the skin and reduce scaly or peeling conditions. Lastly, vinegar regulates the pH of the skin. Vinegar is most effective when used with lavender, rosemary, rose or elder flower. The method could hardly be simpler but it is essential to use top-quality white wine or cider vinegar. Dry any fresh plant material for two days before using.

Measure and mix any dried plant material and then add the vinegar and any blended essential oils (see pages 34 and 37). Cosmetic vinegars composed entirely of liquids can be used at once. Those containing plant material must be left to macerate. Prepare the latter in a screwtop jar and leave on a window sill as instructed, strain and then bottle. To use, add 1 teaspoon of cosmetic vinegar to a cup of still bottled water to wash your face or pour 3–4 tablespoons into a bath.

LAVENDER, ROSEMARY AND ROSEWOOD

VINEGAR	500ml (17½fl.oz) good-quality white wine or cider vinegar
ESSENTIAL OILS	3ml lavender, 3ml rosemary and 2ml rosewood
PLUS	2 tablespoons glycerine

CALENDULA AND ELDER FLOWER

PLANT MATERIAL	50g (1¾oz) calendula flowers and 75g (2⅔oz) elder flowers
VINEGAR	1 litre (2 pints) good-quality white wine or cider vinegar
MACERATE	2 weeks

LAVENDER, ROSE, PINK AND LIME

PLANT MATERIAL	30g (1oz) each of lavender flowers, rose petals, pinks and lime flowers
VINEGAR	1 litre (2 pints) good-quality white wine or cider vinegar
MACERATE	2 weeks

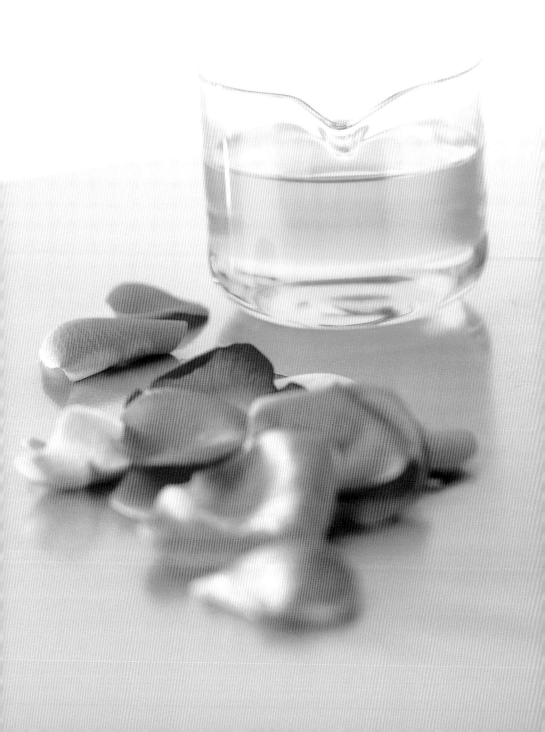

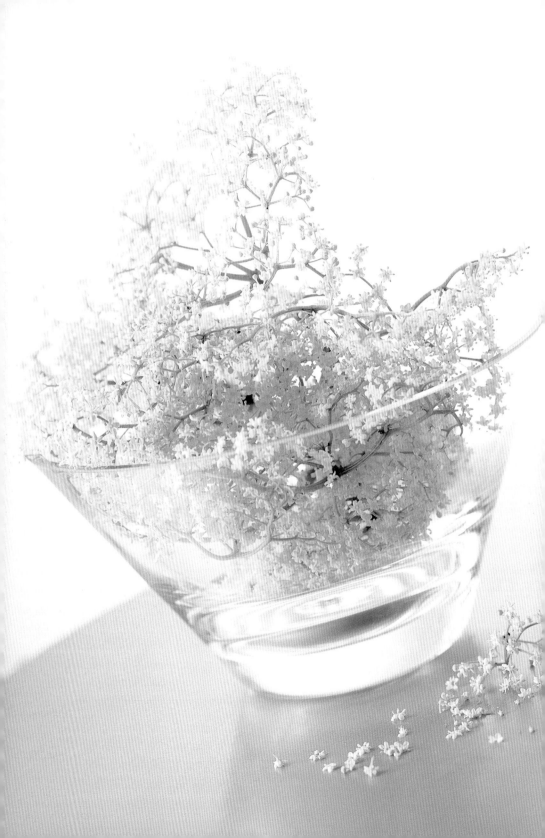

cleansing

recipes

traditional almond milk

The use of almond milk for the skin can be traced back to the Egyptian pharoahs. As beneficial today as it was then, this gentle lotion nourishes as it cleanses. Almonds contain a variety of trace elements, vitamins A and B, and oleic and linoleic acids (or vitamin F), two of the polyunsaturated fatty acids which are vital for healthy skin. Honey boosts the nourishing effect with additional trace elements and enzymes. Throw away any left over after a week.

INGREDIENTS
50g (1¾oz) ground almonds
2 tablespoons organic honey
500ml (17½fl.oz) still bottled water

METHOD
Add the ground almonds and honey to the bottled water and stir well until the honey has dissolved. Leave to rest for 2 hours. Filter, pour into a covered container or bottle and store in a refrigerator.

Apply generously to the face and neck, using a cottonwool ball, and leave for approx. 20 minutes – time for the lotion to penetrate the skin and dry naturally.

EFFECT	cleanses, nourishes
SKIN TYPES	all, especially dry and ageing
FREQUENCY OF USE	twice daily
SHELF LIFE	1 week in refrigerator
PREPARATION TIME	10 minutes, plus 2 hours' resting time
TREATMENT TIME	20 minutes

clay and witchhazel eye mask

This astringent mask is particularly useful for the fragile skin around the eyes. To use on the face and neck, multiply all the quantities by three, and see page 29 for application and removal. For hydrolats, see page 45; for clay, see pages 22–24.

INGREDIENTS

1 tablespoon witchhazel hydrolat
1 tablespoon cornflower hydrolat
1 tablespoon white or green clay powder
still bottled water

METHOD

Following the basic method described on page 23, add the witchhazel and cornflower hydrolats to the clay and leave to rest for 30 minutes without stirring. Then mix well to make a smooth paste.

Apply a thin layer very gently around the eyes and leave for approx. 10 minutes. Rinse carefully with still bottled water and pat dry.

VARIATION

Substitute rosewater hydrolat for the cornflower for a more toning effect.

EFFECT	cleanses, tones, reduces inflammation
SKIN TYPES	all
FREQUENCY OF USE	twice daily for 2 weeks
SHELF LIFE	8 hours in refrigerator
PREPARATION TIME	10 minutes, plus 30 minutes' resting time
TREATMENT TIME	eyes: 10 minutes; face and neck: 20 minutes

fresh orange juice and clay mask

Orange is the gentlest of the astringent citrus juices. Rich in vitamins B and C, plus calcium, potassium, phosphorus, manganese, copper and zinc, and antioxidants, it is an excellent substitute for water in a clay mask. For clay, see pages 22–24; for hydrolats, see page 45.

INGREDIENTS
1 medium orange
2 tablespoons white or green clay powder
still bottled water
witchhazel hydrolat

METHOD
Slice and press the orange to extract 3 tablespoons of juice. Following the standard method described on page 23, add the orange juice to the clay and leave to rest for 30 minutes before stirring. Then mix thoroughly for a smooth paste.

For application to the face and neck, see page 29. After approx. 20 minutes, rinse off, using still bottled water and cottonwool balls, and pat dry. Dab on witchhazel and leave to dry naturally.

VARIATION
Use grapefruit juice for a more astringent, light bleaching action on freckles or the brown spots of ageing skin.

EFFECT	cleanses, tones
SKIN TYPES	all
FREQUENCY OF USE	daily
SHELF LIFE	6 hours in refrigerator
PREPARATION TIME	10 minutes, plus 30 minutes' resting time
TREATMENT TIME	20 minutes

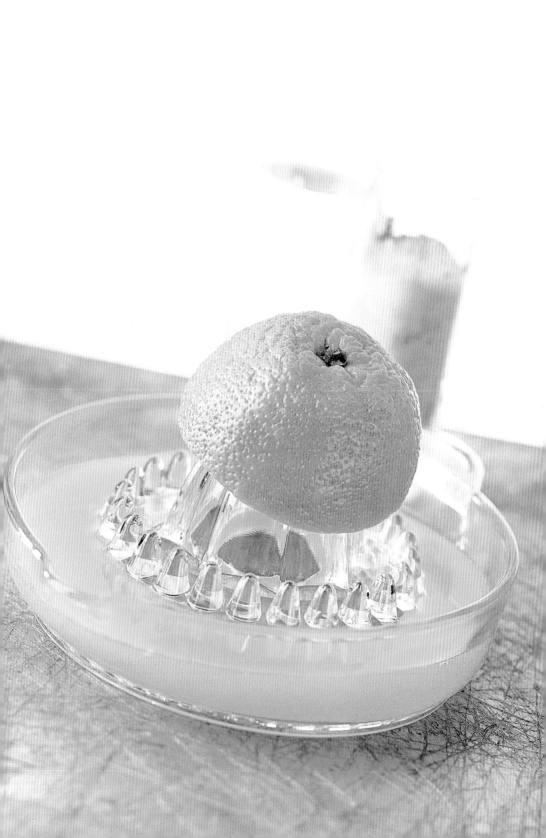

honey and cucumber cleansing milk

This simple recipe cleans the skin while reducing inflammation. The milk contains lactic acid, an excellent natural cleanser with a revitalising, balancing effect on the pH of the skin. The honey is rich in nourishing trace elements, and the cucumber juice hydrates and reduces inflammation. For infusions, see page 30.

INGREDIENTS

¼ small cucumber

2 tablespoons organic honey

1 tablespoon fresh full-cream milk

still bottled water or chamomile infusion

METHOD

Peel and deseed the cucumber. Purée the flesh, using a food processor or blender, and extract 2 tablespoons of juice by sieving through a piece of muslin. Stir the honey into the juice. Once they are well mixed, add the milk and stir again.

Apply the lotion evenly to the face and neck, using cottonwool balls. Leave for approx. 20 minutes before rinsing off with still bottled water or a chamomile infusion and cottonwool balls. Pat dry.

EFFECT	cleanses, reduces inflammation, nourishes, hydrates
SKIN TYPES	all
FREQUENCY OF USE	once or twice daily
SHELF LIFE	6 hours in refrigerator
PREPARATION TIME	5 minutes
TREATMENT TIME	20 minutes

clay and cucumber cleansing mask

A fast-acting cooler for inflamed skin, this recipe is especially useful for eczema and rosacea. The astringent grapefruit juice is both bleaching and toning. For clay, see pages 22–24; for hydrolats, see page 45; for infusions, see page 30; for carrier oils, see pages 34 and 38.

INGREDIENTS
½ **medium cucumber**
½ **grapefruit**
2 tablespoons white or green clay powder
still bottled water
rosewater hydrolat or chamomile infusion

METHOD
Peel and purée the cucumber in a food processor or blender and then strain through a piece of muslin, reserving 2 tablespoons of juice. Extract 1 tablespoon of juice from the half grapefruit. Following the clay mask method described on page 23, substitute the cucumber juice and grapefuit juice for the water and leave to rest for 30 minutes without stirring before mixing to a smooth paste.

For application to the face and neck and removal, see page 29, rinsing off with still bottled water. Finish with rosewater hydrolat or an infusion of chamomile and leave to dry naturally.

VARIATION
For a dry skin, drop the grapefruit juice and stir 1 tablespoon of sweet almond oil into the smooth paste.

EFFECT	cleanses, reduces inflammation, tones
SKIN TYPES	all (see VARIATION for dry skin)
FREQUENCY OF USE	once or twice a week
SHELF LIFE	8 hours in refrigerator
PREPARATION TIME	10 minutes, plus 30 minutes' resting time
TREATMENT TIME	20 minutes

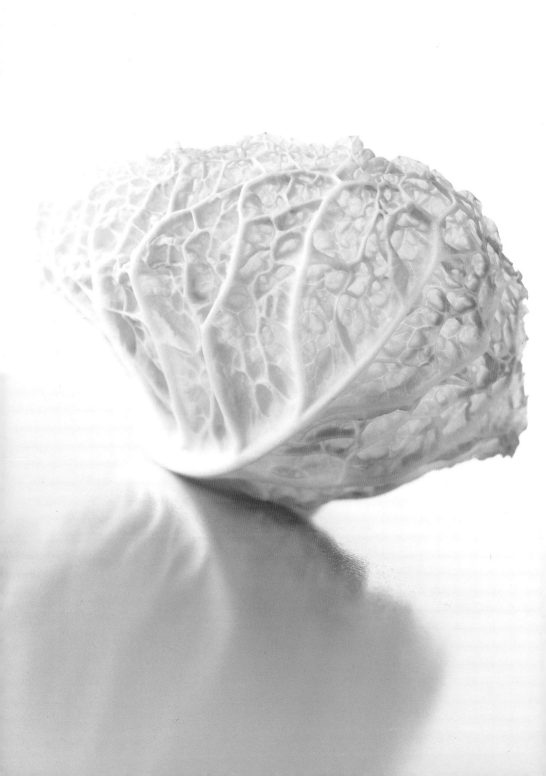

fresh cabbage leaf cleanser

The virtues of the cabbage – rich in vitamins A, B, C, E and K, potassium, sulphur and copper – have been known for thousands of years. Its vegetable acids and minerals have a deeply cleansing effect. This mask is particularly good for acne, eczema or overexposure to wind or sun. For carrier oils, see pages 34 and 38; for hydrolats, see page 45.

INGREDIENTS

¼ **small green cabbage**

1 large carrot or 2 tablespoons fresh carrot juice

½ **lemon**

1 tablespoon olive oil

2 tablespoons white or green clay powder

still bottled water

rosewater hydrolat

METHOD

Discard the outer leaves of the cabbage. Chop the remainder, rinse, and pat dry. If making your own carrot juice, prepare 2 tablespoonsful. Press the lemon to extract 1 teaspoon of juice. Combine the cabbage, carrot juice, lemon and olive oil in a blender or food processor and whizz to a smooth purée. Add 3 tablespoons of the purée to the clay powder and stir to mix.

Apply to the face and neck and leave for approx. 20 minutes. Remove with still bottled water and cottonwool balls and pat dry. Dab on a little rosewater, and leave to dry naturally.

EFFECT	cleanses, heals, anti-inflammatory
SKIN TYPES	all
FREQUENCY OF USE	once a week, or daily for inflamed or damaged skin
SHELF LIFE	24 hours in refrigerator
PREPARATION TIME	10 minutes
TREATMENT TIME	20 minutes

white or green clay cleansing milk

This cleanser has a very slightly drying action, which makes it particularly suitable for use on oily or combination skin. For clay, see pages 22–24; for infusions, see page 30.

INGREDIENTS

1 tablespoon white or green clay powder
250ml (8¾fl.oz) still bottled water

METHOD

Simply add the clay to the bottled water and store in a covered container or bottle in the refrigerator.

Shake before use and apply evenly to the face, neck and hands, using cottonwool balls. Leave for approx. 20 minutes to penetrate the skin and dry naturally.

VARIATION

For an anti-inflammatory effect, use a chamomile infusion instead of bottled water.

EFFECT	cleanses
SKIN TYPES	normal, oily, combination
FREQUENCY OF USE	twice daily
SHELF LIFE	1 week in refrigerator
PREPARATION TIME	5 minutes
TREATMENT TIME	20 minutes

rosewater and lemon juice cleanser

Lemon juice is a very effective cleanser and toner. The most powerful astringent of the citric fruit acids, it also contains vitamin B3 or PP (a strong astringent), which inhibits bacterial action on the skin. In this recipe lemon toughens up rosewater's gentler balancing and tonic action. Good-quality hydrolat is essential; it is now widely available from specialist shops and by mail order (see page 126). For more about hydrolats, see page 45.

INGREDIENTS
½ **lemon**
100ml (3½fl.oz) rosewater hydrolat

METHOD
Press the lemon to extract 1 teaspoon of juice and simply add to the rosewater. Store in a covered container or bottle in the refrigerator.

Apply twice a day to the face and neck, using cottonwool balls. Transfer to a spray bottle if you prefer to mist the skin. Leave to penetrate and dry naturally.

EFFECT	cleanses, tones
SKIN TYPES	oily, combination
FREQUENCY OF USE	twice daily
SHELF LIFE	1 week in refrigerator
PREPARATION TIME	2 minutes
TREATMENT TIME	20 minutes

fresh milk and tomato juice cleanser

Good tomatoes are an abundant source of vitamins A, B (including folic acid) and C, potassium and magnesium, plus valuable antioxidants and trace elements. The high acid content in the recipe – lactic acid in the milk, and fruit acid in the tomato – gives this cleansing lotion a gentle peeling action. Test on the inside arm or wrist for any possible allergic reactions before using on the face. For infusions, see page 30.

INGREDIENTS

1 medium very ripe tomato

approx. 150ml (5¼fl.oz) fresh full-cream milk

still bottled water or chamomile infusion

METHOD

Pulp the tomato, using a food processor or blender. Strain through a piece of muslin and reserve the juice. Add to it an equal amount of milk. Store in a covered container or bottle in the refrigerator.

Apply to the face and neck, using cottonwool balls, once or twice a day. Leave on for approx. 10 minutes and remove with still bottled water or an infusion of chamomile and pat dry.

EFFECT	cleanses
SKIN TYPES	oily, combination (but test first, see above). Not recommended for sensitive skin.
FREQUENCY OF USE	once or twice daily for 1 week
SHELF LIFE	6 hours in refrigerator
PREPARATION TIME	5 minutes
TREATMENT TIME	10 minutes

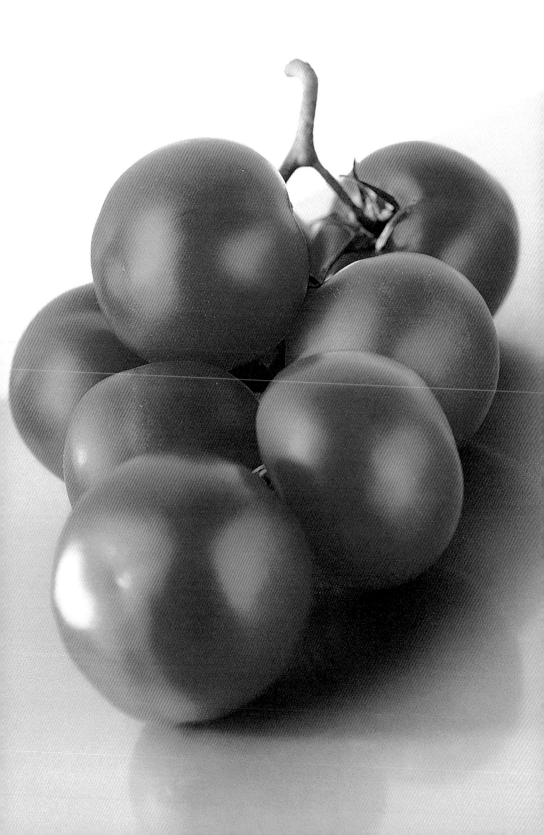

rosewater and witchhazel cleanser

A traditional cleansing recipe, this one also has a strong toning action. Applied lightly around the eyes, it helps to reduce the faint lines of expression that begin to appear in the mid 20s. But take care – hydrolats contain distilled essential oils and even in this form they can make your eyes sting if carelessly applied. It can also be used as a general toner on ageing skin. For hydrolats, see page 45.

INGREDIENTS

200ml (7fl.oz) rosewater hydrolat

100ml (3½fl.oz) witchhazel hydrolat

METHOD

Measure the rosewater and witchhazel into a bottle, close tightly and shake well to mix. This preparation can be kept for several weeks and there's no need to store it in a refrigerator.

Apply carefully twice a day, using cottonwool balls. Leave for approx. 20 minutes to dry naturally.

EFFECT	cleanses, tones, reduces inflammation
SKIN TYPES	all (see above)
FREQUENCY OF USE	twice daily
SHELF LIFE	1 month
PREPARATION TIME	2 minutes
TREATMENT TIME	20 minutes

lime and orange blossom cleanser

Orange blossom is particularly good for dry skin, and lime flowers for ageing skin. Here they combine with cider vinegar's regulating effect on the pH of the skin and its tonic action on the tiny blood vessels that serve the dermis, in a recipe that vitalises as it cleanses. For more about vinegar, see page 46; for hydrolats, see page 45.

INGREDIENTS

1 tablespoon dried lime flowers
50ml (1¾fl.oz) cider vinegar
150ml (5¼fl.oz) orange blossom hydrolat

METHOD

Place the lime flowers in a small bowl and pour on the cider vinegar to cover. Leave to soak for 1 hour. Strain, reserving the vinegar, and add to the orange blossom hydrolat. Store in a closed brown glass bottle.

Apply to the face and neck, using cottonwool balls, and leave to dry naturally.

VARIATION

Substitute elder flower for the lime flower. The effect is similar, although elder flower is also recommended for inflamed skin.

EFFECT	cleanses, tones, balances pH
SKIN TYPES	all
FREQUENCY OF USE	once or twice daily
SHELF LIFE	1 month
PREPARATION TIME	5 minutes, plus 1 hour's soaking time
TREATMENT TIME	10 minutes

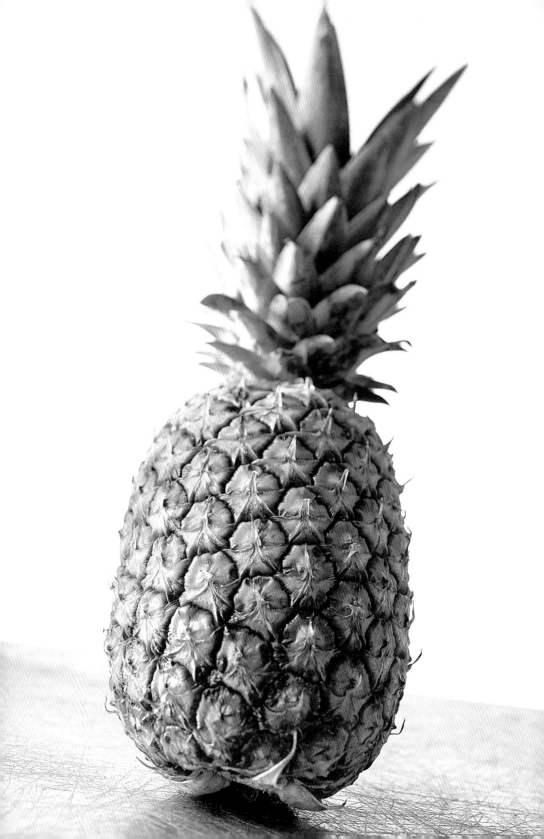

pineapple exfoliating mask

An excellent way to use the tougher, sometimes inedible, central section of the fruit, this mask acts as a gentle peeling agent. Pineapple is rich in vitamins A, B (including folic acid) and C, potassium, magnesium, manganese, iron and sulphur, plus a particularly effective combination of citric and malic fruit acids and enzymes. Although it may irritate a sensitive skin slightly, allergic reactions to pineapple are rare and the chamomile infusion and anti-inflammatory oatmeal will counteract the effect. For infusions, see page 30.

INGREDIENTS
1 ripe medium pineapple
1 cup chamomile infusion, cooled
2–3 tablespoons oatmeal
still bottled water

METHOD
Peel the pineapple and cut it in half lengthways. Remove the pithy central section, using a knife or spoon, and purée it in a food processor or blender. Stir 2 tablespoons of chamomile infusion into the purée, mixing well, and then enough oatmeal to make a smooth paste.

Apply to the face and neck, avoiding the area around the eyes, and leave for approx. 15 minutes. Remove with still bottled water, using cottonwool balls. Dab on some of the remaining chamomile infusion and leave to dry naturally.

EFFECT	cleanses
SKIN TYPES	all (see above for sensitive skin)
FREQUENCY OF USE	once a week
SHELF LIFE	12 hours in refrigerator
PREPARATION TIME	5 minutes
TREATMENT TIME	15 minutes

strawberry and almond oil cleanser

Use this recipe to remove makeup, cleanse and tone the skin. The fruit acid in the strawberries acts as a gentle peeling agent and astringent, while the sweet almond oil counterbalances the effect, preventing too aggressive an action. If you have a sensitive skin, test the lotion on the inside arm or wrist. For carrier oils, see pages 34 and 38; for infusions, see page 30.

INGREDIENTS

6 large, very ripe strawberries
2 tablespoons sweet almond oil
still bottled water or chamomile infusion

METHOD

Whizz the strawberries in a food processor or blender to make a thick juice. Add the sweet almond oil and stir to mix well.

Apply to the face and neck and leave for approx. 10 minutes. Rinse off with still bottled water or an infusion of chamomile, using cottonwool balls, and pat dry.

VARIATION

For those who are allergic to strawberries, try raspberries for a similar, but slightly less astringent, effect.

EFFECT	cleanses, tones
SKIN TYPES	normal, oily, combination. See VARIATION if allergic to strawberries.
FREQUENCY OF USE	once daily
SHELF LIFE	12 hours in refrigerator
PREPARATION TIME	5 minutes
TREATMENT TIME	10 minutes

oat and lemon juice mask

Anti-inflammatory oats and soothing almond oil complement lemon's citric acid in a robust, deep-cleansing, astringent mask. Its tonic action is especially good for preventing moisture loss in ageing skin. For carrier oils, see pages 34 and 38; for hydrolats, see page 45; for infusions, see page 30.

INGREDIENTS

1 lemon (or orange for normal skin)
2 tablespoons sweet almond oil
4 tablespoons porridge oats
witchhazel hydrolat (as required)
still bottled water
rosewater hydrolat

METHOD

Slice and press the lemon or orange to extract 3 tablespoons of juice. Stir the lemon juice and sweet almond oil into the oats. Then gradually add enough witchhazel to make a smooth paste, stirring all the time.

Apply evenly to the face and neck and leave for approx. 15 minutes. Remove, using still bottled water and cottonwool balls, and pat dry. Dab on a little rosewater, leaving to dry naturally.

VARIATIONS

For a more nourishing effect, substitute olive oil for sweet almond oil. Use an infusion of chamomile instead of witchhazel for a less astringent effect.

EFFECT	cleanses, tones, reduces inflammation
SKIN TYPES	all, especially ageing
FREQUENCY OF USE	once a week
SHELF LIFE	12 hours in refrigerator
PREPARATION TIME	5 minutes
TREATMENT TIME	15 minutes

papaya exfoliating lotion

An enzyme called papain, most abundant in the flesh of the unripe papaya, acts as an excellent mild exfoliant – literally digesting dead skin cells. The chamomile infusion should counteract the potential for inflammation. But if you have a sensitive skin or are prone to allergic reactions, test first on your inside arm or wrist. Finishing with rosewater rather than chamomile has a more toning effect. For infusions, see page 30; for hydrolats, see page 45.

INGREDIENTS
1 large fresh papaya
1 cup chamomile infusion, cooled
still bottled water
rosewater hydrolat (optional)

METHOD
Peel the papaya, remove the seeds and purée the flesh in a food processor or blender. Press through a piece of muslin to extract all the juice. Mix the juice with an equal amount of chamomile infusion, stirring well.

Using cottonwool balls, apply the lotion to the face and neck, avoiding any contact with the eyes. Leave for approx. 10 minutes and rinse off with still bottled water. Dab on a little of the remaining chamomile infusion or some rosewater and leave to dry naturally.

VARIATION
Dabbing with papaya juice is an excellent way to remove blackheads.

EFFECT	cleanses
SKIN TYPES	all, but test if sensitive or prone to allergic reactions
FREQUENCY OF USE	once a week
SHELF LIFE	12 hours in refrigerator
PREPARATION TIME	10 minutes
TREATMENT TIME	no more than 10 minutes

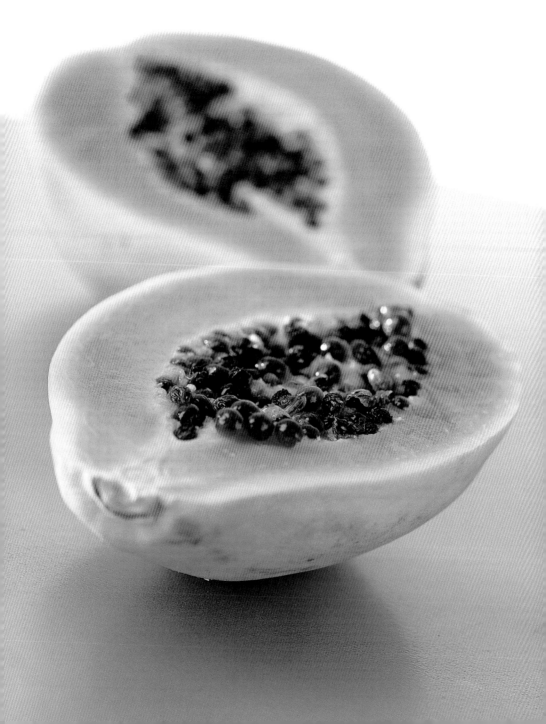

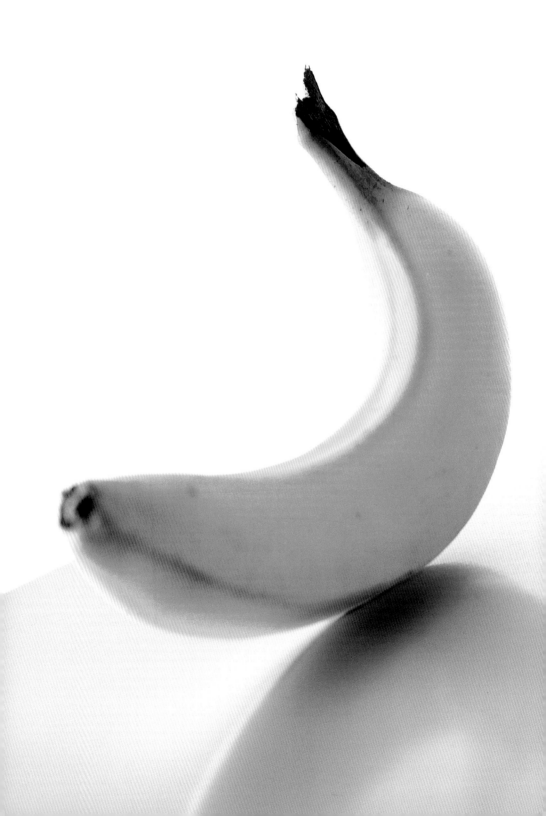

banana anti-ageing mask

Bananas are one of the most nourishing fruits available because they contain large quantities of magnesium, potassium, iron, zinc and iodine, and vitamins A, B (folic acid), E and F. Here they are teamed with double cream (traditionally used to prevent wrinkles) and organic honey in a recipe crammed full of nutrients. For hydrolats, see page 45.

INGREDIENTS

1 small banana
approx. 2 tablespoons fresh double cream
1 tablespoon organic honey
approx. 1 tablespoon potato flour
still bottled water
rosewater hydrolat

METHOD

Mash the banana, using the back of a fork, and then add 2 tablespoons of fresh double cream, the honey and 1 tablespoon of potato flour. Stir to mix well. You may need to add a little more cream or potato flour to obtain the consistency of thick cream or yoghurt.

Apply the mask to the cleaned face, including the area around the eyes and the neck, and leave for approx. 30 minutes. Rinse off with still bottled water and cottonwool balls and dab on a little rosewater, leaving to dry naturally.

EFFECT	nourishes
SKIN TYPES	dry, ageing
FREQUENCY OF USE	3 times a week
SHELF LIFE	6 hours in refrigerator
PREPARATION TIME	5 minutes
TREATMENT TIME	30 minutes

geranium oil and clay mask

This wonderfully scented mask derives its richness from the high vitamin E content in wheatgerm oil and the linoleic acid (or vitamin F) in evening primrose oil, while geranium oil has a balancing, hydrating effect on the skin. Rosewood's gentle tonic action combines with the clay to make this recipe astringent as well as nourishing. For oils, see pages 34–41; for clay, see pages 22–24; for hydrolats, see page 45.

INGREDIENTS

1 tablespoon wheatgerm oil

2 capsules evening primrose oil (contents only)

3 drops rosewood essential oil

3 drops geranium essential oil

3 tablespoons white or green clay powder

3 tablespoons rosewater hydrolat

still bottled water

METHOD

Blend the wheatgerm and evening primrose carrier oils and then combine with the blended rosewood and rose geranium essential oils (see page 37). Add to the clay. Pour on the rosewater and leave for 30 minutes before stirring. Mix well into a smooth paste.

For application to the cleaned face and neck, see page 29 and leave for approx. 20 minutes. Remove with still bottled water and cottonwool balls.

EFFECT	nourishes, cleanses, tones, reduces inflammation
SKIN TYPES	all, but avoid during first 3–4 months of pregnancy
FREQUENCY OF USE	once a week
SHELF LIFE	12 hours in refrigerator
PREPARATION TIME	5 minutes, plus 30 minutes' resting time
TREATMENT TIME	20 minutes

spirulina vitalising mask

The blue-green algae called spirulina are rich in beta-carotene and trace elements very beneficial to an ageing or damaged skin. You will find spirulina in powder form in most health-food shops. When applied daily, this mask is also effective in the treatment of acne. For clay, see pages 22–24; for carrier oils, see pages 34 and 38; for hydrolats, see page 45.

INGREDIENTS

1 tablespoon spirulina powder

2 tablespoons white or green clay powder

1 tablespoon olive oil

still bottled water

rosewater hydrolat

METHOD

Add the spirulina to the clay and stir in the olive oil. Pour on 3 tablespoons of still bottled water and leave for 30 minutes without stirring. Then mix well to make a smooth paste.

For application to the cleaned face and neck, see page 29. Leave for approx. 20 minutes and then wash off with still bottled water, patting dry with cottonwool balls. Dab on a little rosewater and leave to dry naturally.

VARIATION

Add 1 teaspoon of royal jelly to the smooth paste to boost the nourishing, vitalising effect.

EFFECT	nourishes
SKIN TYPES	all
FREQUENCY OF USE	once a week
SHELF LIFE	8 hours in refrigerator
PREPARATION TIME	5 minutes, plus 30 minutes' resting time
TREATMENT TIME	20 minutes

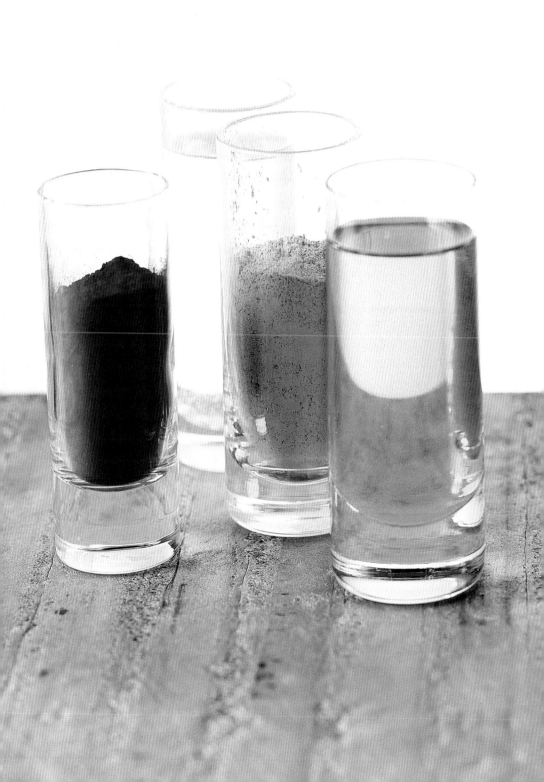

yoghurt and carrot juice mask

This is an excellent mix for improving the elasticity of a dry skin. The yoghurt has a good balancing effect on the pH. Carrot contains precious rejuvenating minerals, and honey's moistening action is invaluable for a tired skin. For carrier oils, see pages 34 and 38; for hydrolats, see page 45.

INGREDIENTS

1 large carrot or 1 tablespoon carrot juice
approx. 2 tablespoons live organic yoghurt
1 tablespoon sweet almond oil
1 tablespoon organic honey
still bottled water
rosewater hydrolat (optional)

METHOD

If making your own carrot juice, prepare 1 tablespoonful. An alternative, if you don't have a juicer, would be to use grated carrot, in which case you need 2 tablespoonsful. Mix the live yoghurt with the carrot, and stir in the sweet almond oil and honey.

Apply to the cleaned face and neck and leave for approx. 20 minutes. Remove with still bottled water and pat dry. Finish with a dab of rosewater left to dry naturally, if you wish.

VARIATION

Use wheatgerm oil instead of sweet almond oil for an even more nourishing effect. Wheatgerm contains vitamin E, which has a powerful healing, regenerative action.

EFFECT	nourishes, balances pH
SKIN TYPES	all, especially dry, ageing or damaged
FREQUENCY OF USE	once a week
SHELF LIFE	6 hours in refrigerator
PREPARATION TIME	5 minutes
TREATMENT TIME	20 minutes

fresh milk and lemon mask

You need fresh full-cream milk for this mask, which helps to balance the pH of a dry or ageing skin. The lemon juice is astringent, and therefore toning, but it also supplies a little vitamin C. For hydrolats, see page 45.

INGREDIENTS
½ lemon
250ml (8¾fl.oz) fresh full-cream milk
rosewater hydrolat

METHOD
Extract the juice of the half lemon and add to the milk, stirring to mix thoroughly.

Apply the resulting mixture to the cleaned face and neck, using cottonwool balls, and leave to penetrate the skin. When the skin is dry, after approx. 20 minutes, clean gently, using rosewater and cottonwool balls. Leave to dry naturally.

EFFECT	nourishes, cleanses, tones, balances pH
SKIN TYPES	all, especially dry or ageing
FREQUENCY OF USE	once daily for 10 days
SHELF LIFE	6 hours in refrigerator
PREPARATION TIME	5 minutes
TREATMENT TIME	20 minutes

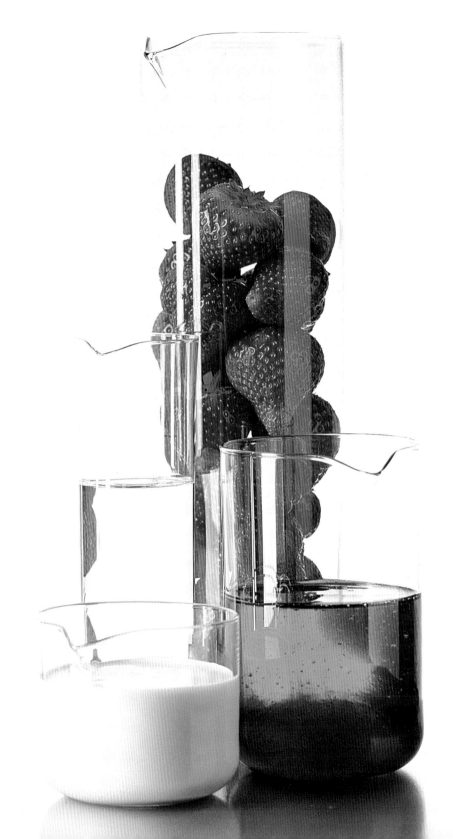

strawberry and cream mask

The honey, with its many trace elements, combines with the cream to nourish tired skin and prevent it from drying too quickly. The salicylic acid in the strawberries cleanses by removing impurities and dead cells. If you have sensitive skin, see page 60. For hydrolats, see page 45.

INGREDIENTS
3–4 medium-sized, ripe strawberries
1 tablespoon fresh double cream
1 tablespoon organic honey
rosewater hydrolat

METHOD
Mash the strawberries with the back of a fork or purée them in a food processor or blender. Add the cream and honey to the purée to form a thick mixture. Add a little more cream if the mixture is too runny, or 1 teaspoon of clay.

Apply to the cleaned face and neck, avoiding the area around the eyes, and leave for approx. 10 minutes. Rinse off, using bottled water and cottonwool balls, and finish with a little rosewater, leaving it to dry naturally.

VARIATIONS
Substitute live yoghurt for the cream to balance the pH of the skin. You can also use raspberries instead of strawberries. The yoghurt/raspberry variation is suitable for sensitive skin, and it is also less likely to cause minor irritation for anyone allergic to strawberries.

EFFECT	nourishes, cleanses, balances pH if you substitute live yoghurt
SKIN TYPES	all (see VARIATIONS for sensitive skin)
FREQUENCY OF USE	once a week
SHELF LIFE	6 hours in refrigerator
PREPARATION TIME	2 minutes
TREATMENT TIME	10 minutes

pollen and egg yolk mask

Pollen and egg yolk are both rich in many of the vitamins, minerals, trace elements and amino-acids needed for a healthy skin. This recipe is particularly beneficial if applied regularly to an ageing or damaged skin. For hydrolats, see page 45.

INGREDIENTS
1 tablespoon unprocessed pollen grains
2 large egg yolks
still bottled water
rosewater hydrolat

METHOD
Pulverise the pollen grains in a food processer or blender with just a few short bursts. You need a fine powder but it is important to avoid heating the pollen because that destroys some of its active ingredients. Add the egg yolks, stirring well to mix.

Apply this mixture to the cleaned face and neck and leave for approx. 20 minutes. Rinse off with still bottled water, using cottonwool balls, and pat dry. Dab on a little rosewater and leave to dry naturally.
VARIATION
You could use 2 tablespoons of fresh double cream instead of the egg yolks. The effect would be similar.

EFFECT	nourishes
SKIN TYPES	all, especially ageing or damaged
FREQUENCY OF USE	once or twice a week
SHELF LIFE	6 hours in refrigerator
PREPARATION TIME	5 minutes
TREATMENT TIME	20 minutes

almond and egg white mask

Nourishing vitamins, fatty acids, trace elements and enzymes in almond and honey combine with the astringent action of egg white to make a very effective mask for dry or ageing skin. For hydrolats, see page 45.

INGREDIENTS

50g (1¾oz) almonds
1 large egg white
1 tablespoon organic honey
rosewater hydrolat (as required)
still bottled water

METHOD

Blanch the almonds in boiling water for 4 minutes and leave to cool. Beat the egg white lightly. Peel the almonds and give them a brief buzz in a blender or coffee grinder until you have a coarse granular texture. Add the lightly beaten egg white and the honey, and blend again to form a smooth paste. If the consistency is too thick to spread easily, stir in some rosewater, a little at a time.

Apply evenly to the cleaned face and neck and leave for approx. 20 minutes. Remove with still bottled water, using cottonwool balls, and pat dry. Dab on a little rosewater and leave to dry naturally.

VARIATIONS

Ground almonds would shorten the preparation time. Finish with a half-and-half mixture of rosewater and witchhazel (see page 62) for a more toning action.

EFFECT	nourishes
SKIN TYPES	dry, ageing
FREQUENCY OF USE	once daily
SHELF LIFE	6 hours in refrigerator
PREPARATION TIME	5 minutes
TREATMENT TIME	20 minutes

honey and egg yolk mask

Egg yolk contains vitamins A, D and E, plus essential amino-acids, minerals and trace elements, in a form which the skin can easily absorb and process. Here it is paired with moisturising honey in a recipe which is an excellent boost for any kind of tired skin. For clay, see pages 22–24; for hydrolats, see page 45.

INGREDIENTS
1 tablespoon organic honey
1 large egg yolk
1 teaspoon white or green clay powder or potato flour
still bottled water
rosewater hydrolat

METHOD
Combine the honey, egg yolk and clay or potato flour, stirring to create a fine paste.

Apply evenly to the cleaned face and neck and leave for approx. 20 minutes. Rinse off with still bottled water, using cottonwool pads, and pat dry. Dab on a little rosewater and leave to dry naturally.

EFFECT	nourishes
SKIN TYPES	all, especially dry or ageing
FREQUENCY OF USE	2 or 3 times a week for dry or ageing skin; once every 2 weeks for remainder
SHELF LIFE	6 hours in refrigerator
PREPARATION TIME	5 minutes
TREATMENT TIME	20 minutes

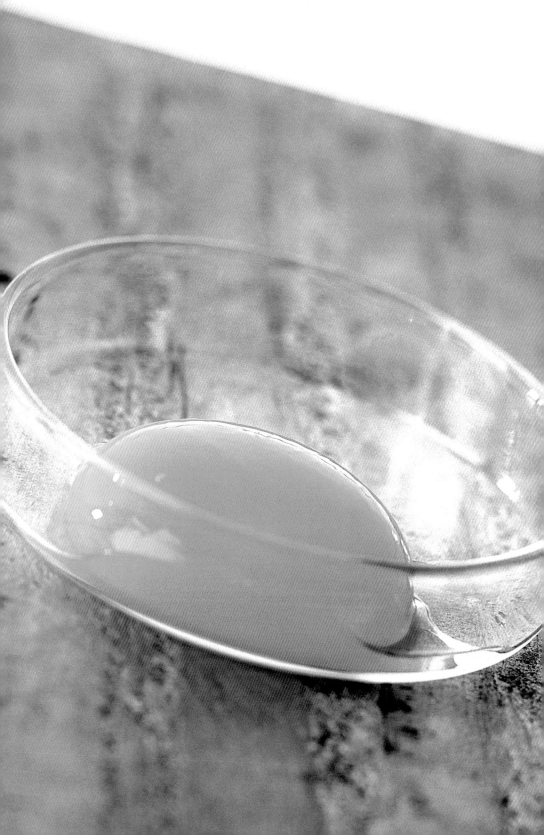

fresh parsley mask

Fresh parsley adds vitamins A, B, C and iron to this toning and nourishing mask, which is particularly good for the neck. Choose double cream for a more nourishing effect on dry skin, yoghurt for other skin types. For oils, see pages 38–39; for hydrolats, see page 45.

INGREDIENTS

1 small bunch fresh parsley
3 tablespoons fresh double cream or live organic yoghurt
1 tablespoon organic honey
2 capsules evening primrose oil (contents only)
still bottled water
rosewater hydrolat

METHOD

Clean the parsley in cold water and remove as much of the stalks as possible. Chop the leaves finely by hand or using a processor or blender. Add the double cream or yoghurt and the honey and evening primrose oil. Stir or blend to mix well.

Apply evenly to the cleaned face and neck and leave for approx. 20 minutes. Remove, using still bottled water and cottonwool pads, and pat dry. Apply a little rosewater and leave to dry naturally.

VARIATIONS

For dry, scaly eczema, use 2 capsules of borage oil instead of primrose oil. For a much stronger anti-inflammatory action, substitute watercress for the parsley.

EFFECT	nourishes, cleanses, tones, reduces inflammation
SKIN TYPES	all, especially ageing
FREQUENCY OF USE	once a week
SHELF LIFE	6 hours in refrigerator
PREPARATION TIME	10 minutes
TREATMENT TIME	20 minutes

avocado and cream mask

This extremely rich mask is packed full of vitamins: avocados alone contain A, B and C, plus essential amino-acids. For carrier oils, see pages 34 and 38; for hydrolats, see page 45.

INGREDIENTS

½ **very ripe avocado**

2 **tablespoons fresh double cream**

1 **tablespoon wheatgerm oil**

3 **capsules evening primrose oil (contents only)**

still bottled water

rosewater hydrolat

METHOD

Peel the stoned, halved avocado and mash the flesh with the back of a fork. Add the double cream, wheatgerm oil and evening primrose oil, stirring well to mix.

Apply evenly to the cleaned face and neck and leave for approx. 20 minutes. Rinse with still bottled water and cottonwool balls and pat dry. Dab on a little rosewater and leave to dry naturally.

VARIATION

Substitute evening primrose oil for 3 capsules of borage oil for a similar but more potent effect.

EFFECT	nourishes
SKIN TYPES	dry, ageing
FREQUENCY OF USE	twice a week for dry skin; daily for ageing skin
SHELF LIFE	6 hours in refrigerator
PREPARATION TIME	5 minutes
TREATMENT TIME	20 minutes

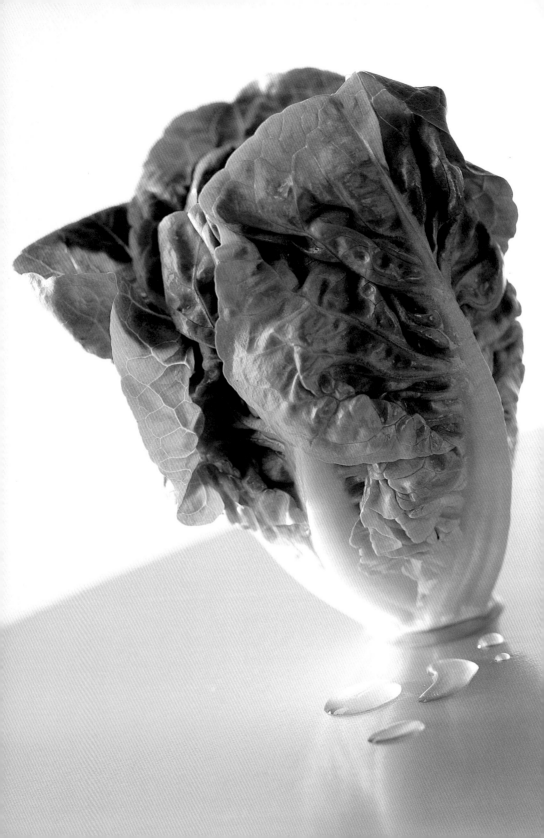

lettuce leaf mask

Cooling and anti-inflammatory, lettuce leaves calm skin rashes and sunburn rapidly, while their vitamins (A, C, D, E and F), precious minerals and trace elements hydrate as well as nourish.

INGREDIENTS
1 very fresh small lettuce, preferably organic

METHOD
Separate the leaves of the lettuce and clean. Toss into boiling water for 5 minutes until cooked. Drain quickly, reserving both leaves and liquid, and allow to cool. The cooking water can be stored in a covered container in the refrigerator and used as a lotion for the face and neck.

Carefully apply the cooled leaves to the cleaned face and neck and leave in place for 5–10 minutes, if possible; they will be rather slippery! Pat the face dry with cottonwool balls.

VARIATION
Purée the cooked lettuce leaves in a food processor or blender. Into the purée stir 3 tablespoons of white or green clay and 1 tablespoon of fresh carrot juice; then add 2 tablespoons of the lettuce cooking water and leave to rest without stirring for 30 minutes. Mix well to form a smooth paste. Apply evenly to the cleaned face and neck and leave for approx. 20 minutes, rinsing off with still bottled water. This makes an excellent mask for dry or ageing skin that suffers from inflammation or dry eczema.

EFFECT	nourishes, hydrates, reduces inflammation
SKIN TYPES	dry, damaged (see also VARIATION)
FREQUENCY OF USE	once daily
SHELF LIFE	cooked leaves: 12 hours in refrigerator; cooking water: 3 days in refrigerator
PREPARATION TIME	10 minutes; VARIATION 10 minutes, plus 30 minutes' resting time
TREATMENT TIME	10 minutes; VARIATION 20 minutes

high nutrient and vitamin mask

Carrot's high vitamin and mineral content – vitamins A and B (folic acid), plus iron, potassium, magnesium, manganese, sulphur and copper – make it an important vegetable in skin care. Here it is teamed with vitamin E (in the wheatgerm) and nourishing honey and yoghurt, in a mask most suitable for those with dry or ageing skin but which can be used occasionally on all types. For carrier oils, see pages 34 and 38; for clay, see pages 22–24; for hydrolats, see pages 14–19 and 45.

INGREDIENTS
1 large carrot or 2 tablespoons carrot juice
approx. 5 tablespoons wheatgerm oil
2 tablespoons organic honey
2 tablespoons live organic yoghurt
1 teaspoon potato flour or clay powder (as necessary)
still bottled water

METHOD
If making your own carrot juice, prepare 2 tablespoonsful. Combine the wheatgerm oil, honey, yoghurt and carrot juice, stirring well. Adjust the consistency by adding a little more wheatgerm oil or carrot juice if too thick, or clay or potato flour if too runny.

Apply evenly to the cleaned face and neck and leave for approx. 20 minutes. Remove with still bottled water and cottonwool balls and pat dry. Dab on a suitable hydrolat and leave to dry naturally.

EFFECT	nourishes, balances pH
SKIN TYPES	all
FREQUENCY OF USE	daily for ageing or damaged skin; once a week for dry skin; 3–4 weeks for other skin types
SHELF LIFE	6 hours in refrigerator
PREPARATION TIME	5 minutes
TREATMENT TIME	20 minutes

healing mask

These blended oils make an excellent mask to apply daily for a few weeks on an ageing or damaged skin, but dry or sensitive skin will benefit too. This quantity will last for about two weeks. For oils, see pages 34–41.

INGREDIENTS

20ml (4tsp) wheatgerm oil

20ml (4tsp) rosehip oil

6 capsules evening primrose oil (contents only)

10 drops geranium essential oil

still bottled water

METHOD

Pour the wheatgerm, rosehip and evening primrose oils into a 50ml (3tbsp) brown bottle (see page 37) and then add the geranium essential oil. Close the bottle and shake well.

Twice a day, dampen the cleaned face and neck lightly with still bottled water and, using a piece of cottonwool, apply a little oil to the entire surface, including the areas around the eyes. Add a little more in any areas which are particularly wrinkled or dry. Don't be overgenerous – only a slight oily film should be left on the skin. Leave it to be absorbed in its own time – it will take approx. 20 minutes. Makeup can be applied as soon as the oil has disappeared.

VARIATION

Substitute borage oil for evening primrose oil. Its effect is more potent.

EFFECT	nourishes
SKIN TYPES	ageing, damaged, dry, sensitive; avoid during first 3–4 months of pregnancy
FREQUENCY OF USE	twice daily
SHELF LIFE	1 month
PREPARATION TIME	5 minutes
TREATMENT TIME	20 minutes

yoghurt and evening primrose mask

Vitamin E and the gamma linoleic acid (or polyunsaturated fatty acid) in evening primrose oil feature strongly in a revitalising mix which must be used for several weeks for best results. For carrier oils, see pages 34 and 38; for clay, see pages 22–24; for hydrolats, see page 45.

INGREDIENTS

3 tablespoons live organic yoghurt

2 capsules evening primrose oil (contents only)

1 teaspoon organic honey

2 capsules vitamin E oil (contents only)

white or green clay powder or potato flour (as necessary)

still bottled water

rosewater hydrolat

METHOD

Mix all the ingredients together, stirring well. If the consistency is too runny, add a little clay or potato flour and stir again.

Apply evenly to the cleaned face and neck and leave for approx. 20 minutes. Rinse off, using bottled water and cottonwool balls, and pat dry. Tone the skin by dabbing on a little rosewater and leave to dry naturally.

VARIATIONS

Substitute 2 capsules of borage oil for the evening primrose oil and/or 1 teaspoon of wheatgerm oil for the vitamin E. Borage oil is more potent than evening primrose oil; wheatgerm contains less vitamin E.

EFFECT	nourishes, balances pH, reduces inflammation
SKIN TYPES	all, especially dry or ageing
FREQUENCY OF USE	twice a week or more for ageing skin; occasionally for remainder
SHELF LIFE	6 hours in refrigerator
PREPARATION TIME	5 minutes
TREATMENT TIME	20 minutes

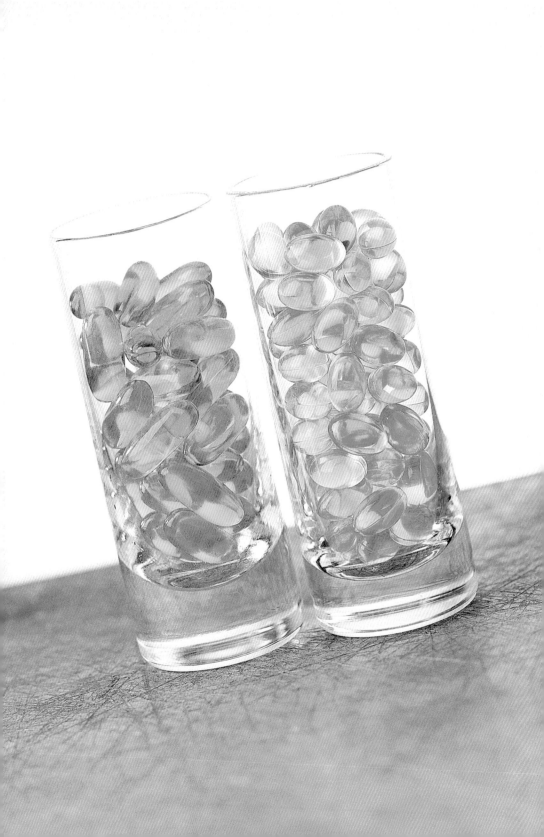

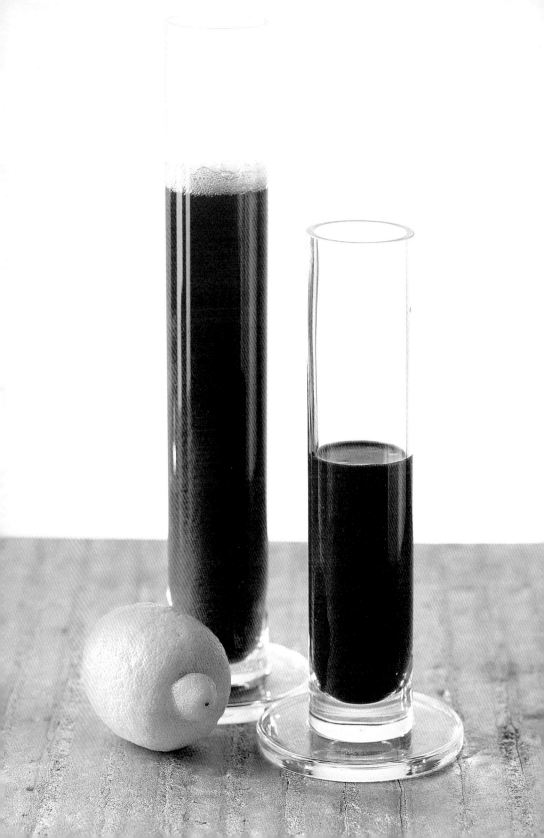

toning and
hydrating
recipes

cucumber and fresh mint mask

The fresh mint and egg white both have a toning action on the skin, while the cucumber is hydrating and anti-inflammatory, making this a mask which can also be used to calm inflamed skin or sunburn.

INGREDIENTS

5 fresh mint leaves
¼ medium cucumber
1 large egg white
still bottled water

METHOD

Place the mint in a food processor or blender and give it one short burst to chop. Peel and deseed the cucumber. Add to the mint in the processor or blender and purée. Beat the egg white until it stands in stiff peaks. Fold it very gently into the puréed cucumber mixture.

Apply evenly to the face and neck and leave for approx. 20 minutes. Rinse off, using still bottled water and cottonwool balls, and pat dry.

VARIATIONS

For an even more toning effect, add 1 teaspoon of freshly squeezed lemon juice or cider vinegar. Trickle slowly into the final mixture, stirring gently all the time.

EFFECT	tones, hydrates, reduces inflammation
SKIN TYPES	all
FREQUENCY OF USE	once a week
SHELF LIFE	6 hours in refrigerator
PREPARATION TIME	10 minutes
TREATMENT TIME	20 minutes

apple juice and clay mask

Substituting fresh apple juice for water in a clay mask creates a more toning preparation for the face and neck. Nourishing wheatgerm counteracts the drying effect of clay on a dry or ageing skin. For carrier oils, see pages 34 and 38; for clay, see pages 22–24; for hydrolats, see page 45.

INGREDIENTS
1–2 apples or 3 tablespoons fresh apple juice
1 tablespoon wheatgerm oil
2 tablespoons white or green clay powder
still bottled water
rosewater hydrolat

METHOD
If making your own apple juice, extract 3 tablespoonsful, using a juicer. Following the clay mask method (see pages 23–24), stir the wheatgerm oil into the clay and pour on the apple juice. Leave to rest for 30 minutes, before stirring to form a smooth paste.

For application to the face and neck and removal, see page 29. Finish with a little rosewater.

EFFECT	tones, cleanses, reduces inflammation
SKIN TYPES	all
FREQUENCY OF USE	once or twice a week
SHELF LIFE	8 hours in refrigerator
PREPARATION TIME	5 minutes, plus 30 minutes' resting time
TREATMENT TIME	20 minutes

egg white and lemon juice mask

This classic recipe is probably still the best toner around, judged for its simplicity and remarkable effectiveness. It is also an excellent treatment for softening the skin of the hands. Egg white's ability to remove impurities and lemon juice's action in inhibiting bacterial growth explain its subsidiary cleansing action. For hydrolats, see page 45.

INGREDIENTS
1 large egg white
½ lemon
still bottled water
rosewater or witchhazel hydrolat

METHOD
Beat the egg white stiffly until it stands up in peaks and press the half lemon to extract 1 teaspoonful of juice. Then simply fold the juice carefully into the egg white.

Apply to the face and neck and leave for approx. 20 minutes. Rinse off, using still bottled water and cottonwool pads, and pat dry. Dab on a little rosewater or witchhazel and leave to dry naturally.

EFFECT	tones, cleanses, nourishes
SKIN TYPES	all
FREQUENCY OF USE	twice a week for ageing skin; once a week for remainder
SHELF LIFE	6 hours in refrigerator
PREPARATION TIME	5 minutes
TREATMENT TIME	20 minutes

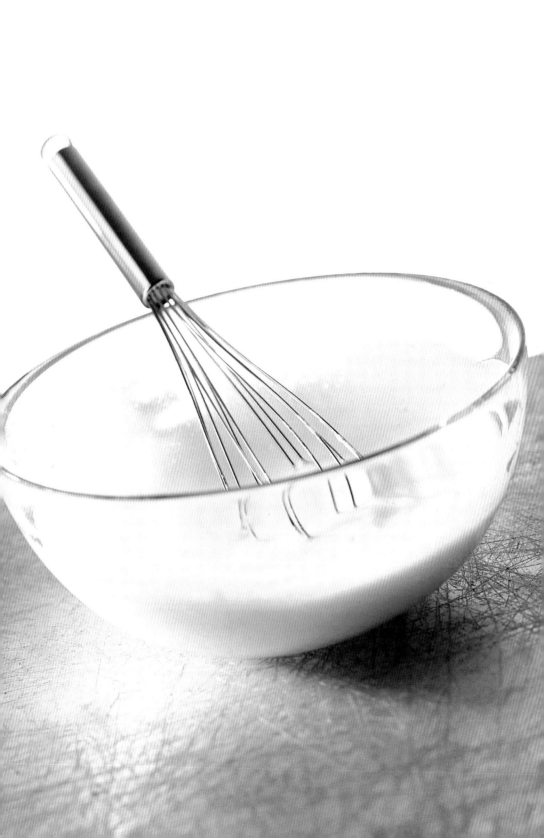

fresh parsley and clay mask

Here astringent witchhazel combines with anti-ageing agents in the fresh parsley and olive oil to make this mask an excellent way to tone and nourish the skin of the neck. It can also be applied to the face, but take care to avoid the eyes. For clay, see pages 22–24; for carrier oils, see pages 34 and 38; for hydrolats, see page 45.

INGREDIENTS
small bunch fresh parsley
2 tablespoons white or green clay powder
3 tablespoons olive oil
2 tablespoons witchhazel hydrolat
still bottled water

METHOD
Wash the parsley in cold water and remove the stalks before chopping the leaves finely by hand or using a food processor or blender. Stir 2 tablespoons of chopped parsley into the clay. Then add the olive oil and witchhazel, and stir again until a thick paste is obtained.

Apply to the neck and jawline and leave for approx. 20 minutes. Rinse off, using still bottled water and cottonwool pads, and pat dry.

VARIATION
Substitute wheatgerm oil for the olive oil if you want the healing, regenerative effect of vitamin E.

EFFECT	tones, nourishes, reduces inflammation
SKIN TYPES	all
FREQUENCY OF USE	once a week
SHELF LIFE	12 hours in refrigerator
PREPARATION TIME	5 minutes
TREATMENT TIME	20 minutes

yoghurt and blackcurrant mask

The fruit acid in blackcurrants is toning, hydrating, cleansing and anti-inflammatory. When complemented with the balancing action of live yoghurt, it creates a mask particularly beneficial for ageing, flushed or inflamed skin. Blackcurrants are also rich in trace elements, minerals (calcium, potassium and magnesium), and vitamins B and C. Use fresh fruit if available, although frozen blackcurrants are acceptable. Avoid canned fruit – it is heated in the preservation process and the juice takes on the properties of purple dye. Removable but hardly relaxing!

INGREDIENTS
4 tablespoons blackcurrants
2 tablespoons live organic yoghurt
still bottled water

METHOD
Crush the blackcurrants in a food processor or blender. Add the live yoghurt to the thick juice and stir well.

Apply to the face and neck and leave for approx. 20 minutes. Rinse off, using still bottled water and cottonwool balls, and pat dry.

EFFECT	tones, cleanses, hydrates, balances pH, reduces inflammation
SKIN TYPES	all, especially ageing
FREQUENCY OF USE	twice a week
SHELF LIFE	6 hours in refrigerator
PREPARATION TIME	5 minutes
TREATMENT TIME	20 minutes

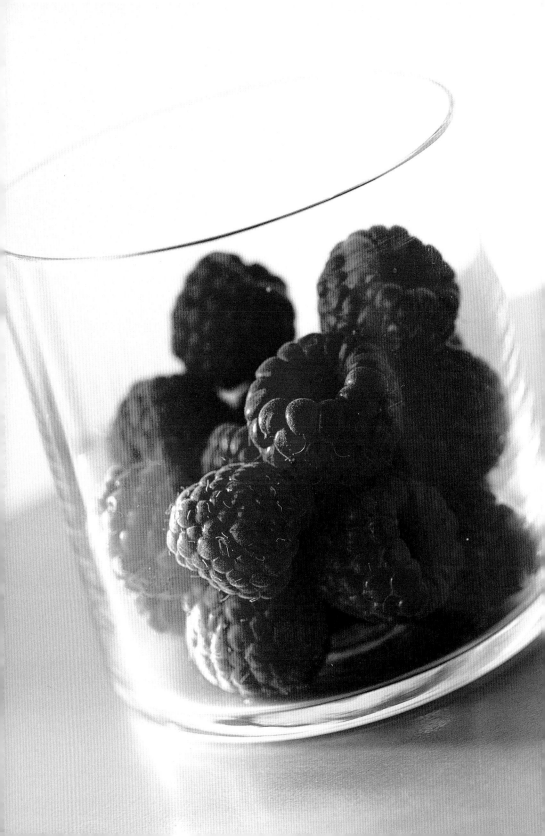

raspberry mask

The three fruit acids (salicylic, citric and malic) in raspberries and the lactic acid in the milk combine for a more astringent, invigorating effect than the blackcurrant mask on page 99. For essential oils, see pages 34 and 40; for hydrolats, see page 45.

INGREDIENTS
approx. 12 raspberries
2 tablespoons fresh full-cream milk
2 drops geranium essential oil
still bottled water
witchhazel hydrolat

METHOD
Using a blender, food processor or fork, crush enough raspberries to obtain 2 tablespoons of purée. Add to it the milk and geranium essential oil, and stir to mix well.

Apply to the face and neck, using cottonwool balls, and leave for approx. 20 minutes. Wipe off, using still bottled water and more cottonwool, and pat dry. Finish by dabbing on a little witchhazel and leave to dry naturally.

VARIATION
For a more balancing effect, substitute live organic yoghurt for the full-cream milk.

EFFECT	tones, hydrates, cleanses, reduces inflammation
SKIN TYPES	dry, combination, and especially ageing
FREQUENCY OF USE	twice a week
SHELF LIFE	6 hours in refrigerator
PREPARATION TIME	5 minutes
TREATMENT TIME	20 minutes

egg white and cucumber mask

This cooling mask is excellent for dry, flushed or inflamed skin. Both the egg white and orange juice have a tonic action, while cucumber is hydrating and anti-inflammatory. Cucumber also contains vitamins A, B and C, plus sulphur, manganese and iodine. For hydrolats, see page 45.

INGREDIENTS
1 large egg white
½ orange
¼ cucumber
still bottled water
witchhazel or rosewater hydrolat

METHOD
Beat an egg white until it forms stiff peaks. Press the half orange to extract 1 tablespoon of juice. Grate enough cucumber to fill 2 tablespoons. Fold the cucumber carefully into the beaten egg white and add the orange juice, stirring gently to mix.

Apply to the face and neck and leave for approx. 20 minutes. Wipe off with still bottled water and cottonwool balls. Then dab on a little witchhazel or rosewater and leave to dry naturally.

EFFECT	tones, cleanses, hydrates, reduces inflammation
SKIN TYPES	dry, combination, ageing, damaged
FREQUENCY OF USE	once or twice a week
SHELF LIFE	6 hours in refrigerator
PREPARATION TIME	5 minutes
TREATMENT TIME	20 minutes

fresh cream and grape lotion

Grapes are rich in minerals (potassium, manganese, calcium, sodium and iodine) and vitamins A, B and C. Black grapes also contain the bioflavonoid quercinine, a powerful antioxidant with an anti-ageing action, so opt for those wherever possible. In this recipe grape and lemon juice act as toners, while the nourishing double cream counterbalances their astringent effect. For hydrolats, see page 45.

INGREDIENTS

several grapes or 1 tablespoon grape juice
½ lemon
1 tablespoon fresh double cream
still bottled water
witchhazel hydrolat

METHOD

If making your own grape juice, crush the grapes with a fork and press through a sieve to extract 1 tablespoonful of juice. Press the lemon to extract half a teaspoonful of juice. Beat the fresh double cream and grape juice together to obtain a light, fluffy cream. Add the lemon juice gradually drop by drop to prevent curdling, stirring gently to mix well.

Apply to the face and neck and leave for approx. 10 minutes. Wipe off, using still bottled water and cottonwool balls. To finish, dab on a little witchhazel and leave to dry naturally.

EFFECT	tones, nourishes
SKIN TYPES	all
FREQUENCY OF USE	once a week
SHELF LIFE	6 hours in refrigerator
PREPARATION TIME	5 minutes
TREATMENT TIME	10 minutes

apple cologne

The malic acid in fresh apple juice is mildly toning, astringent and helps to keep the skin clear, making this recipe suitable even for sensitive skin. It will keep for weeks due to its high alcohol content and is therefore useful when travelling. Good-quality aftershave is even better than eau de cologne because it is likely to contain calming essential oils.

INGREDIENTS

3–4 apples or 100ml (3½fl.oz) fresh apple juice
1 teaspoon sea salt
1 tablespoon organic honey
60ml (2¼fl.oz) good-quality eau de cologne or aftershave

METHOD

If making your own apple juice, prepare 100ml (3½fl.oz) and filter through a paper towel. To the juice, add the sea salt, honey and eau de cologne or aftershave. Pour into a bottle, cover and shake well to mix.

Use twice a day, applying to the face and neck with a cottonwool ball and leaving to dry naturally.

VARIATION

You can substitute filtered grape juice (see page 103) for the apple juice; the effect will be similar.

EFFECT	tones, hydrates, cleanses, nourishes
SKIN TYPES	all
FREQUENCY OF USE	twice daily
SHELF LIFE	1 month
PREPARATION TIME	5 minutes
TREATMENT TIME	20 minutes

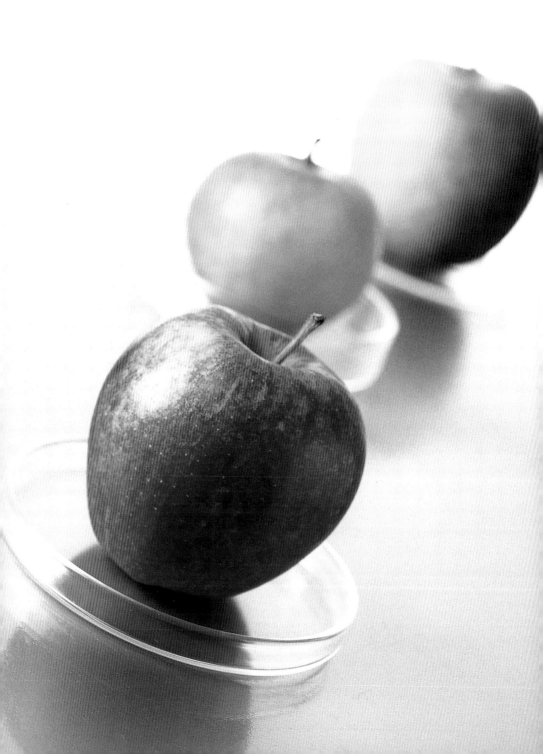

rosewater astringent lotion

The combination of lemon juice, rosewater and witchhazel makes for an astringent toner which needs moisturising, nourishing honey to keep it balanced. Like the previous recipe, this one is a useful travelling companion. Choose aftershave if you want to enhance the soothing action. For hydrolats, see page 45.

INGREDIENTS

½ lemon
50ml (1¾fl.oz) rosewater hydrolat
50ml (1¾fl.oz) witchhazel hydrolat
1 tablespoon organic honey
50ml (1¾fl.oz) eau de cologne or aftershave

METHOD

Press the half lemon to extract 1 teaspoon of juice. Combine the rosewater and witchhazel, and then add the honey, lemon juice and eau de cologne or aftershave, stirring well. Pour into a bottle and cover to store.

Use twice a day, applying to the face and neck with cottonwool balls and leaving to dry naturally.

EFFECT	tones
SKIN TYPES	all
FREQUENCY OF USE	twice daily
SHELF LIFE	1 month
PREPARATION TIME	5 minutes
TREATMENT TIME	20 minutes

cucumber and vinegar lotion

It is the cucumber that hydrates and reduces inflammation. Vinegar and vodka are essentially toners here. This is a speedy recipe if you have cosmetic vinegar to hand. If you don't, turn to page 46 for a description of its properties and how to make it. Incidentally, this is not an opportunity to get rid of that bottle of malt vinegar lurking in your store cupboard. You must use good-quality white wine or cider vinegar.

INGREDIENTS
½ cucumber
cosmetic vinegar
2 tablespoons strong vodka

METHOD
Peel and deseed the cucumber. Using a food processor or blender, pulp the flesh. Extract and reserve all the juice by sieving through a piece of muslin. Add to the cucumber juice an equal amount of cosmetic vinegar and then the vodka, and stir well. Store in a closed bottle in the refrigerator.

Use twice a day, applying to the face and neck with cottonwool balls and leaving to dry naturally.

EFFECT	tones, hydrates, reduces inflammation
SKIN TYPES	all
FREQUENCY OF USE	twice daily
SHELF LIFE	2 weeks in refrigerator
PREPARATION TIME	10 minutes
TREATMENT TIME	20 minutes

barley and rosemary lotion

Rosemary tones, improving blood circulation in the skin. Barley water is a mild cleanser with some nourishing properties: barley contains vitamins B and E, and essential minerals (iodine, potassium, calcium, magnesium, iron and copper). Soaking the barley for 24 hours is not essential but it causes the grain to germinate, releasing a variety of enzymes which constitute an exfoliant gentle enough for sensitive skin.

INGREDIENTS

100g (3½oz) barley
1 litre (1¾pt) water
generous handful fresh rosemary or 3 tablespoons dried rosemary

METHOD

Ideally, cover the barley with cold water and leave it to soak for 24 hours. Reserving the barley, strain off the soaking water. Cook the pre-soaked barley in 1 litre (1¾ pints) of fresh water for 30 minutes, bringing it to the boil, covering and then leaving to simmer. Strain immediately, discarding the barley. Add the rosemary to the cooking water, covering and leaving to infuse until cool. Strain the liquid again and store in a closed bottle in the refrigerator.

Using cottonwool balls, apply twice a day to the face and neck and leave to dry naturally.

EFFECT	tones, cleanses, nourishes, reduces inflammation
SKIN TYPES	all
FREQUENCY OF USE	twice daily
SHELF LIFE	4 days in refrigerator
PREPARATION TIME	40 minutes, plus optional 24-hour 'soaking time'
TREATMENT TIME	20 minutes

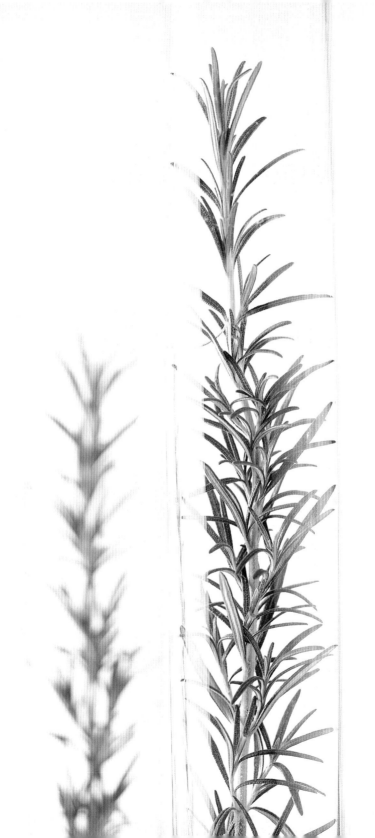

fresh juice toner

This recipe depends for best results on very fresh ingredients. Here highly astringent lemon plays the minor role in a mix of toning fruit acids. For advice on blackcurrants, see page 99; for grapes, see page 103.

INGREDIENTS

½ **cup blackcurrants**

approx. 10 grapes or 75ml (2⅔fl.oz) fresh grape juice

½ **lemon**

METHOD

Crush the blackcurrants in a food processor or blender and strain through a piece of muslin, reserving the juice – you need 75ml (2⅔fl.oz). Repeat with the grapes if making your own grape juice. Press the half lemon to extract 1 tablespoonful of juice. Pour the grape juice and blackcurrant juice into a bottle and add the lemon juice. Cover and store in the refrigerator.

Apply to the face and neck twice a day, using cottonwool balls, and leave to dry naturally.

EFFECT	tones, hydrates
SKIN TYPES	all
FREQUENCY OF USE	twice daily
SHELF LIFE	48 hours in refrigerator
PREPARATION TIME	10 minutes
TREATMENT TIME	20 minutes

rosewater, honey and lemon lotion

This recipe combines the toning effect of rosewater, the nourishing qualities of honey and the potent astringent action of lemon juice. Multiply the quantities given by five and you have enough for a week. For hydrolats, see page 45.

INGREDIENTS

½ **lemon**

2 tablespoons rosewater hydrolat

1 teaspoon organic honey

METHOD

Press the half lemon to extract the juice and mix with the rosewater and honey, stirring well.

Apply daily to the face and neck, using cottonwool balls, and leave to dry naturally.

EFFECT	tones, hydrates, nourishes, cleanses
SKIN TYPES	all
FREQUENCY OF USE	once daily
SHELF LIFE	1 week in refrigerator
PREPARATION TIME	2 minutes
TREATMENT TIME	20 minutes

fresh melon lotion

Melons are cooling and hydrating, being mostly composed of water and natural sugars, plus small amounts of vitamins A, B and C. Indeed, used alone, crushed melon flesh will quickly calm the pain of a mild burn or sunburn. Lemon, the toner, and olive oil are complementary and work together to balance the pH of the skin. For carrier oils, see pages 34 and 38.

INGREDIENTS

¼ **fresh, ripe melon**

½ **lemon**

1 tablespoon olive oil

METHOD

Peel and deseed the melon. Press the half lemon to extract 1 teaspoon of lemon juice. Using a food processor or blender, purée the fresh melon. Filter its juice through a piece of muslin and reserve. Add to the melon juice the olive oil and lemon juice, and store in a covered bottle or container in the refrigerator.

Shake well before use. Apply twice a day to the face and neck, using cottonwool balls, and leave to dry naturally.

VARIATIONS

For a longer lasting but less hydrating preparation, add 2 tablespoons of good-quality eau de cologne or aftershave after the lemon juice.

EFFECT	tones, hydrates, reduces inflammation
SKIN TYPES	all
FREQUENCY OF USE	twice daily
SHELF LIFE	in refrigerator: BASIC RECIPE 48 hours; VARIATIONS: 2 weeks
PREPARATION TIME	10 minutes
TREATMENT TIME	20 minutes

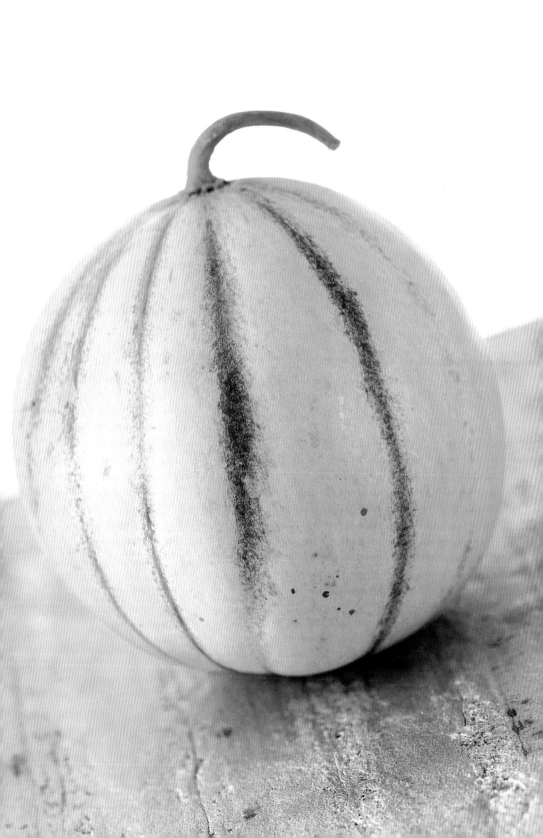

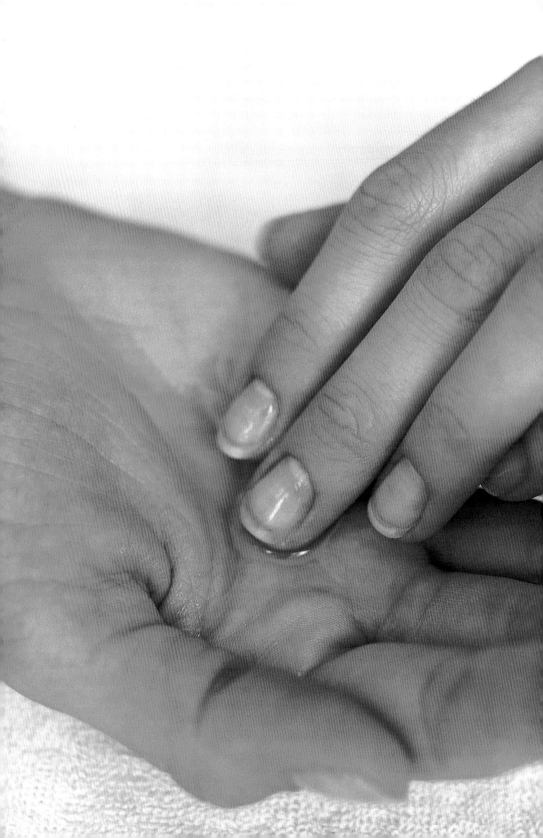

acne

This very common condition affects more females than males. Although it starts in, and is often associated with, teenagers, it can recur for years, sometimes right through to middle age. The characteristic small fatty lumps – actually swollen sebaceous glands (see page 6) – are frequently inflamed and topped with black or white heads, which, if squeezed, can set off a cycle of re-infection due to bacterial activity on the surface of the skin. When the lumps do finally subside, some scarring is almost inevitable. The face is most likely to be affected, but acne can also appear on the neck, shoulders, back and sometimes on the upper chest.

Acne occurs in people whose sebaceous glands are particularly sensitive to testosterone. Known as the male hormone, testosterone is in fact produced in varying amounts by both sexes. Medical research has revealed that there is an increased amount of testosterone in women's skin at the end of each monthly cycle, just before menstruation begins, and this explains why women susceptible to acne often report that it seems to get worse at the same time each month.

Present evidence suggests that changes in eating habits, alterations in stress levels and exposure to sunlight can make acne either better or worse. However, as the cause is predominantly hormonal and hereditary, it is true to say that until it is possible to alter a person's genetic makeup acne is going to remain treatable but not curable.

In susceptible people, even slight exposure to many hair sprays may result in a sudden outbreak of acne. Plastic components in the spray block the larger pores, usually around the mouth, chin and the sides of the face, creating what is called an anaerobic (or no air) environment. Many of the commonplace facial bacteria are low-oxygen organisms and actually thrive in such conditions. So, if you suffer from acne, read the labels on cosmetic and hair products carefully and avoid any that contain synthetic polymers, such as vinyl and other plastics.

Black heads, white heads and spots are all caused to varying degrees by constant hyper-secretion of the sebaceous glands and a number of frequently associated infections.

CONVENTIONAL TREATMENT

The standard treatment consists of regular courses of antibiotics which help to prevent the germs in the small fatty lumps from multiplying.

In very severe cases, vitamin A (or retinoid) acid has been successful in removing all the symptoms of acne, but often only after a severe worsening of the condition. However, this treatment can have serious side effects: among them, the malfunction of the liver, severe rheumatic symptoms with painful inflammation and stiffening of the joints, and high cholesterol. It is strictly forbidden for pregnant women, and patients are warned not to become pregnant for at least three months after treatment has ended. In fact, the effects can be so serious that treatment is available only in hospital: your general practitioner will not be able to provide the regular monitoring that is essential.

ALTERNATIVE TREATMENT

The best alternative to conventional treatments and their long-term side effects is to use essential oils, which are not only antibacterial and anti-inflammatory but are also able to regulate the natural production of sebum. It is, of course, also imperative to keep the skin clean, and steaming is often effective, although there is a risk that it will increase the inflammation. The temptation to squeeze the black or white heads must be resisted. Squeezing only causes further inflammation and scarring. For hydrolats, see page 45; for infusions, see page 30; for oils, see pages 34–44; for steaming, see page 33.

TWICE DAILY

to cleanse Apply a simple cleansing lotion, using 1 part witchhazel hydrolat, 1 part cold chamomile infusion and a few drops of fresh lemon juice. This mix has a shelf life of seven days in a refrigerator so make a week's supply at a time.

to control bacterial activity Massage the affected areas, combining an astringent carrier oil, such as hazelnut, with:

1. one of the antibacterial essential oils: juniper, niaouli or tea tree, and
2. one of the anti-inflammatory oils: chamomile or lavender.

TWICE A WEEK

to deep cleanse and nourish Apply the revitalising clay and spirulina recipe (see page 74). Apart from removing oil, dirt and bacteria very effectively, the clay contains minerals (including iron oxide, calcium and various salts) and trace elements (including copper, magnesium and zinc) to help the natural healing of damaged skin, while spirulina provides the whole spectrum of vitamin A. You can boost this mix by adding 3 drops of chamomile, juniper or niaouli essential oil to the clay before the liquid. Alternatively, just add your essential oil to a simple clay mask (see page 23).

ONCE A WEEK OR MORE

to remove excess oil and open clogged pores Steam, adding a few drops of one of the anti-inflammatory or antibacterial essential oils listed on page 117 or 1 heaped tablespoon of dried chamomile, calendula, thyme or yarrow. This will also help to eliminate redness.

boils

In most cases caused by a bacterial infection, boils are sited in hair follicles. A large, single boil or a tight group of smaller boils develops, with an accumulation of pus, swelling, inflammation and pain.

CONVENTIONAL TREATMENT

A course of antibiotics is the usual prescription. Some scarring may occur, especially if boils reappear in the same place.

ALTERNATIVE TREATMENT

For oils, see pages 34–41; for clay, see pages 22–23; for infusions, see page 30.

TWICE DAILY

to deep cleanse A local application of a basic clay mix will help to eliminate pus, toxins and residual infection; as an alternative to water, substitute cucumber juice or a cold infusion of chamomile.

to reduce pain and inflammation Apply a slice (or the pulp) of a raw potato. Raw cabbage leaf is also very good for reducing inflammation and promoting healing.

to heal Apply neat juniper, niaouli or tea tree essential oil to the infected area, using cottonwool balls, three or four times a day.

AFTER HEALING

to reduce scarring and prevent further infection Using light massage twice daily, apply a mix of equal amounts of rosehip seed and sweet almond carrier oils, blended with 5 per cent of two essential oils: choosing either niaouli or tea tree plus lavender. Alternatively, apply neat vitamin E oil directly onto the scar twice daily.

cracks and fissures

These often appear at the corners of the mouth, the edge of the nostrils and behind the ears, less commonly on the fingers, and are sometimes complicated by fungal or bacterial infections.

CONVENTIONAL TREATMENT

Most people rely on an over-the-counter antiseptic cream.

ALTERNATIVE TREATMENT

For infusions, see page 30; for cosmetic vinegar, see page 46; for oils, see pages 34–41.

TWICE DAILY

to cleanse Bathe the affected areas with half a mug of cool chamomile infusion, mixed with 1 teaspoon of cosmetic vinegar.

to heal Apply locally an oil mix, combining apricot kernel plus 10 per cent vitamin E oil or half-and-half calendula and rosehip seed as the carrier, blended with a healing/astringent essential oil, such as cedarwood or cypress, and one of the following antiseptic essential oils: lavender, lemon, niaouli, rosewood or tea tree. An application of fresh, raw cabbage leaf may also be effective.

damaged skin

The general appearance of skin severely scarred by acne, accident, burns or surgery or thickened due to chronic eczema can often be improved, using a natural skin-care programme. Conventional treatment is non-existent.

ALTERNATIVE TREATMENT

It is essential to cleanse damaged skin well before applying healing oils or masks. Clay masks are particularly useful, and the substitution of freshly pressed pineapple or papaya for water in a standard clay mask greatly increases its action upon the epidermis. For oils, see pages 34–41; for clay, see pages 22–24.

DAILY

to reduce inflammation Vegetable masks are useful. Substitute a cabbage leaf in the lettuce-leaf treatment (see page 87) or simply dab on a half-and-half mix of fresh cabbage and carrot juices. A little clay powder added to the juices as a thickening agent will also make a simple mask; leave it on the skin for 20 minutes before removing with still bottled water and cottonwool balls.

to improve appearance Using a cottonwool ball, apply locally to the slightly dampened skin one of the following oil mixes. (Note: 40 drops of essential oil = 1ml.)

1. Carrier oil: 100ml rosehip seed. Essential oils: 1ml cedarwood, 2ml geranium, 1ml rosewood, 1ml sandalwood.

2. Carrier oils: 50ml rosehip seed, 25ml calendula and 25ml hypericum. Essential oils: 2ml frankincense, 2ml palmarosa, 1ml rosemary. The contents of three capsules each of borage (or evening primrose) and vitamin E may also be added to either.

TWICE A WEEK

to deep cleanse Use a pineapple exfoliating mask (see page 65) or a papaya exfoliating lotion (see page 68). The application of neat papaya juice is a speedier alternative – remove after 5 minutes.

eczema

The condition affects about one person in four. The symptomatic rash is accompanied by swelling, blistering, itching and scaling. Bacteria tend to proliferate in the affected areas, causing the skin to become inflamed, infected and sometimes weepy. Although eczema can be an allergic reaction, the causes are sometimes unknown; some types are thought to be hereditary and are therefore difficult to treat.

CONVENTIONAL TREATMENT

A regimen of antibiotics, anti-inflammatories and cortisone cream is the recommended approach.

ALTERNATIVE TREATMENT

For chronic eczema, consider also the treatment indicated under damaged skin. For oils, see pages 34–41; for clay, see pages 22–24; for infusions, see page 30.

DAILY

to reduce inflammation See damaged skin. Cucumber, potato or watercress juice may be applied directly to the skin, using a cottonwool ball.

to soothe and heal Massage with an oil mix twice daily. The most useful essential oils are the anti-inflammatories, such as chamomile or lavender, and the antibacterial, anti-fungal and anti-viral oils, such as juniper, lemon, niaouli, rosewood and tea tree. Choose two or three essential oils and mix with calendula, hypericum or rosehip seed carrier oil; if the skin is very dry, substitute in the carrier oil(s) 10 per cent each of one or two of the following: borage (or evening primrose oil) and vitamin E.

TWICE A WEEK

to soothe, cleanse and heal Apply a clay mask, using instead of water fresh cucumber, carrot, cabbage, grape or melon juice, or an infusion of chamomile. If the skin is very dry, add 1 tablespoon of olive oil to the mask.

psoriasis

This chronic, hereditary skin condition is characterised by the accumulation of excessive numbers of cells in the epidermis, causing both inflammation and flaking. A complete cure is not possible, but lengthy periods of remission are commonplace.

CONVENTIONAL TREATMENT

Moderate cases are treated with preparations containing coal tar, salicylic acid or zinc, plus psoralen (a molecule which renders the skin more sensitive to UVB rays) accompanied by ultraviolet radiation. In the worst cases, the regular administration of a type of vitamin A acid (acitrecin) is also quite successful in removing all symptoms, but some of the side effects are serious: see the warnings on the effects of another form of vitamin A therapy under acne on page 117. In addition, malfunction of the kidneys has been reported, and pregnancy must not occur during and for two years after the completion of the treatment.

ALTERNATIVE TREATMENT

The sun has a very beneficial effect on a psoriatic skin. Daily massage with a mix of olive oil and the essential oil bergamot often produces a good improvement without significant side effects. Use no more than 1ml of bergamot to 100ml of olive oil. Bergamot is not listed in the essential-oil chart because it contains psoralen, making it unsuitable for more general use (see page 9). For oils, see pages 34–39.

rosacea

At first the sufferer exhibits a mass of tiny red spots on and around the nose and cheeks. Symptoms appear suddenly, accompanied by extreme itching or a burning sensation, subside and then the cycle begins again. At a late stage of chronic rosacea, congestion and even deformity in the affected area (especially of the nose) may occur. Skin affected by rosacea is dry, hot and inflamed, but this condition is often associated with an oily condition of the skin, such as acne or seborrhoeic dermatitis. The cause is unknown.

CONVENTIONAL TREATMENT

The regular use of antibiotics is the most common procedure. One of the vitamin A acids (tretinoid) is also quite successfully employed, but see acne for the side effects. In the worst cases, cosmetic surgery is the only option left. Large amounts of the affected tissues of the nose and surrounding area are removed, which certainly improves the general appearance of the face, but it cannot be done without a certain amount of scarring.

ALTERNATIVE TREATMENT

Rosacea should be treated at the earliest possible stage to obtain the best results. Antibacterial and anti-inflammatory essential oils constitute the best alternative to conventional treatment and its long-term side effects. For oils, see pages 34–41; for infusions, see page 30; for clay, see pages 22–23.

DAILY

to heal and soothe Using an astringent carrier oil, such as hazelnut, combined with calendula or hypericum, and a blend of two essential oils chosen from chamomile, geranium, lavender, palmarosa, rosewood and tea tree, it is possible to regain control over the condition and often cure it. Apply with cottonwool balls, dabbing gently.

to soothe A chamomile infusion may bring quick relief from pain and inflammation. Cabbage, lettuce and watercress are also good for acute inflammation. The cooked leaves can be applied directly to the skin (see page 87) or the juice mixed with an equal quantity of cucumber juice and used as a lotion or substituted for water in a basic clay mask. Alternatively, a purée can be mixed with an equal amount of clay powder, adjusting with more purée or clay (if necessary) for a simple mask.

TWICE A WEEK

to eliminate inflammation Regular application of a cooling clay mask using cucumber juice (see page 55) or a clay lotion, substituting a chamomile infusion for the bottled water (see page 58, VARIATION), is helpful. Do not steam the face.

to cool and soothe Melon and blackcurrant are anti-inflammatory. Use the fresh juice of either mixed with an infusion of chamomile as a calming, soothing lotion, and the pulp with clay as a mask (see *to soothe*, on the previous page).

seborrhoeic dermatitis

This inflammation is caused by hyperactive sebaceous glands (see page 6) and is most commonly found in people with oily or combination skins. It appears first on the forehead and sides of the nose, spreading rapidly to other parts of the face and the scalp. At this stage the sufferer looks sunburnt and, indeed, often experiences a rather unpleasant, burning sensation. Fungal yeast organisms are always present in this type of inflammation.

CONVENTIONAL TREATMENT

Coal tar, zinc and salicylic preparations are usually prescribed for the face and scalp. The condition also responds to anti-fungal preparations but is made considerably worse by the application of cortisone creams.

ALTERNATIVE TREATMENT

Antibacterial and anti-inflammatory essential oils which are able to regulate the production of sebum constitute the best alternative form of treatment. For oils, see pages 34–44; for steaming, see page 33; for clay, see pages 22–23.

TWICE DAILY

to control bacterial or yeast activity Massage, using an astringent carrier oil, such as hazelnut, blended with one of the anti-fungal essential oils, such as niaouli, rosewood or tea tree, and an anti-inflammatory oil such as chamomile or lavender. Recent studies also indicate that the daily application of borage oil is rapidly beneficial in some cases;

apply locally, using a cottonwool ball, or supplement the carrier oil in the recipe above, using no more than 15 per cent of borage oil.

to soothe Cucumber juice and watercress or lettuce will calm acute inflammation. For watercress and lettuce, see *rosacea*.

WEEKLY

to clean clogged pores Regular steaming will remove the excess sebum, and the addition of an anti-inflammatory and antibacterial oil or herb (see page 33) will help to eliminate some of the redness. Do this more than once a week, if possible.

to deep cleanse A basic clay mask is very effective. Apart from removing oils, dirt and bacteria, clay can import minerals and trace elements valuable in the natural healing of a damaged skin. The more powerful fruit masks and lotions, such as pineapple (see page 65) and papaya (see page 68), are also useful.

sunburn

If severe, see a doctor immediately or go to the nearest casualty department; you may require special dressings, antibiotics or treatment for sunstroke.

ALTERNATIVE TREATMENT

For oils, see pages 34–41.

TWICE DAILY

to soothe mild sunburn Dab neat lavender essential oil on the worst affected areas. On other areas, dilute the lavender oil in a half-and-half blend of calendula and olive oil carrier oils, using no more than 5 per cent lavender oil. Applications of raw cabbage or lettuce leaves are also helpful in calming inflammation and reducing the pain. Avoid massage or rubbing and masks of any kind.

However, prevention, as always, is better than cure, especially when you consider that prolonged exposure to the sun is the major cause of prematurely aged skin. For sun and the skin, see pages 8–11.

list of suppliers

✉ Indicates that a mail-order service is available.

ACUMEDIC LIMITED ✉
101–5 Camden High Street,
London NW1 7JN
tel: 020 7388 6704
fax: 020 7387 5766
web: http://www.acumedic.com.
Natural skin-care range,
books on TCM and natural
medicine

AROMANTIC ✉
22 Drumine Road, Forres,
Scotland IV36 1HX
tel: 01309 676600
e-mail: aromantic4@aol.com
Natural cosmetic products,
oils and clay

ATAR AROMATHERAPY
95–7 North Main Street,
Wexford, Eire

tel and fax: 00353 5321 755
Oils and other natural
products

P.J. COUSIN HERBAL
AND COSMETIC SUPPLIES
Kensington Health Centre,
211–213 Kensington High Street,
London W8 6BD
tel: 020 7376 1199
e-mail: pjc@cousin.sonnet.co.uk
Advice and oil mixes, top-
quality organic oils, hydrolats
and herbs

NEAL'S YARD REMEDIES ✉
26–34 Ingate Place,
Battersea, London SW8 3NS
tel: 020 7498 1686
fax: 020 7478 2055
e-mail:mail@nealsyardremedies.com

Oils, natural cosmetic products,
nutritional supplements and
herbs

NUTRICENTRE ✉
7 Park Crescent, London
W1N 3HE
tel: 020 7436 5122
e-mail: enq@nutricentre.com
web:http://www.nutricentre.co.uk
Vitamin and nutritional
supplements, oils, clay and
other natural products

PLANET ORGANIC
42 Westbourne Grove,
London W2 5SH
tel: 020 7221 1345
Oils, vitamin supplements
and natural products

SHIRLEY PRICE
AROMATHERAPY LIMITED ✉
Essentia House,
Upper Bond Street,
Hinckley, Leicestershire
LE10 1RS
tel: 01455 615466
fax: 01455 615054
e-mail: shirleypricearoma@
compuserve.com
Top-quality oils and natural
cosmetics, aromatherapy
and beauty equipment

TISSERAND
AROMATHERAPY ✉
Newtown Road, Hove, East
Sussex BN3 7BA
tel: 01273 325666
fax: 01273 208444
web: www.tisserand.com
Full range of essential oils

index

ACKNOWLEDGEMENTS

The photographs of all recipe ingredients were taken by Diana Miller and styled by Wei Tang. All other photographs, of massage and masks, were taken by Graham Atkins Hughes and the masks and massage movements were modelled by Flavia Eberhard from Models One.

Publisher's Note

Please note that although this book includes recommended treatments for particular skin conditions, they are not substitutes for regular medication and treatment. We recommend that you consult your doctor before trying any of the treatments, particularly if you are pregnant or have a medical condition. Whilst every care has been taken in compiling this book, no responsibility can be accepted by the author or the publishers for any consequence resulting directly or indirectly from the use or adaptation of any of the contents of this book, or from any omission from it.

First published in 2001 by
Quadrille Publishing Limited, Alhambra House,
27–31 Charing Cross Road, London WC2H 0LS

This paperback edition first published in 2002

© Text Pierre Jean Cousin 2001
© Design and layout Quadrille Publishing Limited 2001

Publishing Director: Anne Furniss
Consultant Art Director: Helen Lewis
Design Assistants: Sarah Emery and Katy Davis
Project Editor: Nicki Marshall
Editor: Mary Davies
Production: Sarah Tucker

British Library Cataloguing in Publication Data
A catalogue record for this book is available from the British Library.

ISBN 1 903845 47 5

Printed and bound by Dai Nippon Printing, Hong Kong